FIT2 FAT 2FIT

The Unexpected Lessons from Gaining and Losing 75 lbs on Purpose

DREW MANNING
WITH BRAD PIERCE

HarperOne
An Imprint of HarperCollins*Publishers*

This book contains advice and information relating to health care. It is not intended to replace medical advice and should be used to supplement rather than replace regular care by your doctor. It is recommended that you seek your physician's advice before embarking on any diet or other health plan. All efforts have been made to assure the accuracy of the information contained in this book as of the date of publication. The publisher and the author disclaim liability for any medical outcomes that may occur as a result of applying the methods suggested in this book.

HarperOne

HarperCollins books may be purchased for educational, business, or sales promotional use. For information please e-mail the Special Markets Department at SPsales@harpercollins.com.

HarperCollins website: http://www.harpercollins.com

FIRST HARPERCOLLINS PAPERBACK EDITION PUBLISHED IN 2013

Designed by Terry McGrath

Library of Congress Cataloging-in-Publication Data is available upon request.

ISBN 978–0–06–219421–3

13 14 15 16 17 RRD(H) 10 9 8 7 6 5 4 3 2 1

CONTENTS

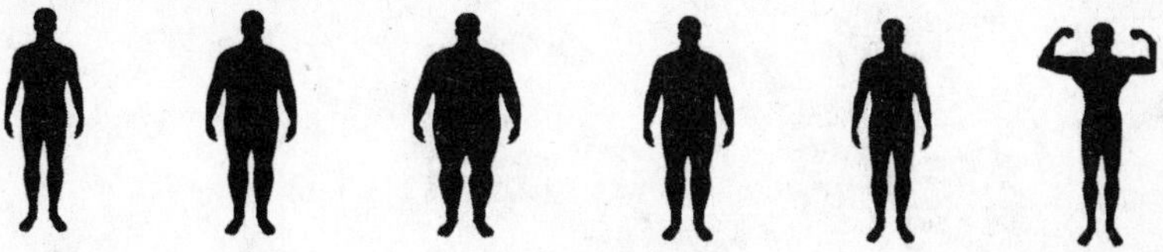

PART ONE

FIT2FAT

FIT2FAT2FIT

CHAPTER 1

EXPECT THE UNEXPECTED

It's the snoring that does it. Lately, it seems to be the snoring that always wakes me up.

Almost out of habit, I glance over my shoulder to my wife's side of the bed, unsurprised to see it empty. I wonder how long she lasted through the tumult before retreating to quieter recesses of the house. My stomach growls loudly, matching the volume of the now-echoing snores that filled the house moments before, and I know it's time to start the day.

These days it takes a strategic combination of momentum and gravity to move from the bed to a standing position. The next steps of my routine fall quickly into place: the staggered walk to the bathroom, followed by brushing my teeth just outside the view of the mirror, and then a shower, a shave, and the lengthy process of getting dressed.

I realize that I need new pants; the elastic on the waist of my current pair is stretched to its maximum. I sit on the corner of the bed, ready for the forced exhale as I try to tie my shoes. Even though I live through this each day, I'm still caught off guard by being out of breath. I used to play full football games with greater ease and stamina, and I'm already dreading the trek down the 12 stairs to the kitchen, though my stomach is protesting with every second of delay. By accident, I see my newly round image in the mirror. Caught by a strange mix of depression and acceptance, I reflect on how and why this happened. And as clearly as the slightly alarming reflection stares back at me, I realize I've become the physical poster child of stereotypes I've spent a lifetime trying to avoid.

There are certain stereotypes men are branded with that are probably a bit unfair. Insinuations that we have the emotional depth of a kiddie pool, consider our, ahem, needs before those of certain other individuals, and believe half the weekends of the year are our own personal opportunity to sit like a couch potato in front of the TV (for the sake of football, of course) are unfair to say the least. Sure, you have your bad eggs out there. But to paint us all with a broad brush is selling our gender short.

However, some gender stereotypes are undeniably true, and regarding these, we men can be painted with the broadest of brushes. Chief among them, and the cause of much of my current angst, is asking for directions. I'm not sure why, but men, in general, think they can get themselves from Point A to Point B by divine intervention. Lick a finger, stick it in the air to determine the direction of the wind, and we're off. We can find our own way. We *must* find our own way.

This is why the idea of a global positioning system (GPS) shakes all men to the core. First of all, a GPS device in a car tells the driver where to go; it doesn't suggest. It dictates every turn, stop, and change in direction. Second, it seems that the voice is always female. In my limited experience with an actual GPS device, I find myself taking the extra step of doubting the instructions *she* provides. I follow instructions initially as the disembodied voice tells me to turn left, turn right, go straight, but then I suddenly start thinking, *How the hell did I end up here?* I purposefully ignore the fact that the GPS will probably tell me to take a few more careful turns and I'll end up where I'm supposed to be. That's beside the point. I'm convinced that men, as a gender, are hardwired with a GPS in the brain. It's the only logical explanation for why we react so poorly when direction or help is provided.

Today I feel like my "inner GPS" dropped me off in the wrong part of the neighborhood, and I have serious doubts about my ability to get home unscathed. It's unnerving to feel this lost in the one area of my life where I always knew the route.

It's hard to believe while looking in the mirror, but I'm a personal trainer. And within that profession, my inner GPS used to provide easy directions—keep going straight. In fact, it's safe to say that long before becoming a personal trainer, I was so devoted to my chosen route that I was addicted—to exercise, and to having large muscles and six-pack abs. I was such a health addict that I invited the opportunity to both judge and attempt to help individuals who weren't born with the "health-nut gene."

Sadly, we live in a society with an ever-expanding waistline. It is estimated that one in three Americans is overweight. Yet, despite all of the potential health-related vices surrounding me, my waist remained trim, my muscles toned. And my attitude—especially my attitude—stood resolute. Anyone struggling with weight could, and should, drop the pounds. It was a choice; the ability to step away from the doughnut, the extra-large french fries, and the comfortable couch was within all of us, not the select few.

Whether I was working with an obese person who medically had to lose weight if he wanted to continue living, or a woman who could stand to lose the 15 pounds of baby weight long after pregnancy, the goal was the same. Get them to see that they were doing this to themselves. Then show them how to think, act, and live differently.

I wish I could say that the results were always stellar, that I always exhibited a strong enough will to show people the error of their ways, and that I managed to create my own breakthrough moments with such people every day. Were there successes? Absolutely. Certain clients listened to me, saw that I was trying to help, and acted on my advice. But more often than not, the response I got was less positive; many clients were full of doubt that I was truly there to help them overcome their struggles. They saw me as someone who didn't get it: I didn't understand how hard it was to set aside the food or how difficult it was to go to the gym and try to do 10 biceps curls while surrounded by prima donna–type gym rats. I didn't understand that weight loss was much more than overcoming the "physical."

For a long time, I rationalized that this was just part of the problem. They were looking for someone to blame for their plight. As they saw it, it wasn't their fault they were overweight; it was society, emotion, self-esteem, and people like me—people who just didn't understand.

Back then I believed that losing weight and getting fit were about simple choices. In this way, I was my clients' worst nightmare—the picture of what they wanted to be, with all the judgment they already had about themselves as to why they were overweight and unhealthy. Yet now I can often be found sitting on our couch, which has perfectly molded itself to my XXL butt, eating Zingers and Pringles as if I were personally keeping both brands afloat.

I decided to do something that, let's face it, most personal trainers will never do. I accepted the small possibility that maybe my clients were right and I was wrong.

I'm overweight. I'm unhealthy. I've started to think that my wife finds me as attractive as a dung beetle. Either that or she considers me to be an extra-squishy sofa, permanently added to our living room furniture. And the strangest part is that it was my choice. I made a decision that I honestly question a little each day. I decided to stop exercising, stop eating healthy, stop being me. I made the decision to embrace the habits I had spent years trying to eradicate.

I decided to do something that, let's face it, most personal trainers will never do. I accepted the small possibility that maybe my clients were right and I was wrong. Maybe I didn't get where they were coming from. After all, my idea of a treat was to have an extra glass of a spinach shake. My idea of a lazy day was cutting my workout by 10 minutes because I needed to go mow the lawn at a full sprint. But what if I was the problem? What if becoming fit and healthy wasn't as simple as saying to yourself, "I'm going to be healthy now"?

I decided to take a journey from fit to fat, and back to fit again. If my message of health and personal accountability wasn't sinking in with my clients, maybe I didn't get how hard the road from unhealthy to healthy really was. Maybe the trainer in me needed to learn a few lessons first. So I made the commitment to spend six months without exercise, living a restriction-free diet. I would force myself to become overweight. Then, after half a year of eating all the typical American foods that feed our desire for convenience more than our need for health and moderation, I would switch gears. I'd put myself through the rigor and pain I'd been trying to get my clients to embrace. I hoped to inspire them to change and take control of their own health.

Yet at this moment, having overachieved in the initial transition from fit to fat, I feel lost. My personal GPS has dropped me at the corner of Shock and Terror. I've gained 75 pounds, which is bad enough. Worse yet, my personality is not the same. I'm full of self-doubt, believing that everyone around me is judging my newfound body type. More than anything, though, I'm afraid.

What if I can't lose the weight? I used to be convinced that I could actually scare fat off my body if I flexed hard enough. Then again, I had expected to gain only 50 pounds on this journey, and here I was at 75. I never knew that those same processed foods I had committed to fighting each day would develop such a stranglehold, both on my psyche and my waistline. And if the pounds *do* come off, will my skin firm up? Will my body process calories at the same pace it did for the first 30 years of my life, or will it be permanently skewed? My head is swirling with thoughts of the effects this experiment has had on my metabolism and the body I worked so tirelessly to perfect.

I used to judge people who couldn't step away from the Cinnamon Toast Crunch. Now, anytime I don't pull the box out of the pantry, I feel like I'm cheating on the little baker captured on the front of the box. If I decide not to hang out with Toucan Sam and his rainbow hoops of pure love and affection, the guilt multiplies. And as a show of support, followers of my journey send me cakes, pies, and other contraband. My guess is that a stalk of celery sent from a well-wisher would not have the same endearing value.

We all struggle with self-esteem, and it would be inaccurate to imply that even on my most fit days I didn't have twinges of self-doubt. But nothing is as extreme as what I feel at my heaviest. These days, I question my abilities as a personal trainer, husband, friend, and father. What if my current reality becomes my permanent reality? Okay, perhaps this is a bit melodramatic, but the fear is real.

I know that I won't allow myself to remain 75 pounds overweight once I have the chance to eat right and work out. But what will the long-lasting effects of this journey be? Will I inherit a pesky 15 pounds that refuse to go away? Will my health be permanently affected?

I wonder whether my wife thinks that now is the time to upgrade to a slimmer, more manicured model. Sure, I'm worried about the weight going away. But I'm downright terrified that my personality, confidence, and self-belief will never be the same. It's still hard to believe that this entire thing was my idea.

CHAPTER 2

WINNERS VS. LOSERS AND OTHER ASSUMPTIONS

One more try. Those were the words that ran through my head as I took a half breath, half sigh, and pushed open the gym door to work with James, a recent client. As I walked past the equipment, filled with individuals either working toward or perfecting sculpted bodies, I went over my new strategy for James.

I barely had enough time to go through the basic points of the speech I was preparing when I saw him standing against the mirrors. He hadn't noticed me yet; he was staring at other people in better shape than he was. Was I imagining it, or was there a sense of resignation in his stare?

As always, I had tried to be encouraging, especially at first, offering comments about how he could get the results he was looking for and change himself and his habits for the long term. By now, though, I knew that I was simply trying to fill the space before his discouragement won out and he would officially quit. As expected, my initial comments had gone over like a lead balloon; James hadn't lost pounds, inches, or his self-doubt. It was now time to make him see that he could change, and that *he* was holding his own health back.

My interactions with James didn't start like this—with me giving unconvincing pep talks to both of us. None of my personal training experiences did. After all, I was obsessive about my own health, and had been for as long as I could remember. I had the biceps and abdominal muscles to prove it: working out and eating right were key parts of who I was, and this "healthy obsession" had led me to become a part-time personal trainer. (I also had a "day job" as a neuromonitoring technician in a hospital.)

Personal training allowed me to share my passion with others, helping them find health and fitness when they'd lost it or if they'd never had it in the first place. Their results gave my life a greater purpose. To be honest, it also got me more time in the gym without making my wife worry that I had a secret cot in the back, adorned with a gold nameplate reading Drew's Place.

After I became a certified personal trainer, friends and family would approach me. Some wanted general advice on surviving the holidays. Others asked for specific exercises that could help them "bulk up," or "lose the last 15 pounds" after pregnancy. Which brings us back to James—a relative who'd approached me with a specific need.

James wasn't just overweight. At 5'8" and 340 pounds, James's physique was now a medical problem. Whereas many people hope to lose a "few" extra pounds, James had to lose weight. If he didn't, the consequences would be much more severe. He'd struggled with extra pounds for most of his life, but a motorcycle accident some time back had damaged his knees, and with that injury came more weight. James wanted help, and I was immediately interested in helping. After some measured success with other individuals, I was ripe for a big success story. Plus, this was family, and James's situation had clearly graduated beyond wanting to shed a little weight—he needed help. If nothing else, if I helped my wife's relative I'd store away Husband of the Year credits for times when I was being the typical, problematic male.

So we hatched a plan for me to become his personal trainer. I would guide him in exercising and provide meal plans to turn his health around. And although I warned him that I could be militant, I also promised to be supportive.

Early on, James followed my meal plans faithfully, and although he often seemed to be on the verge of cursing me during our workouts, he pushed himself every time. We were working out three times a week, and the level of effort he made impressed me. Even better, the weight started to come off. Granted, it wasn't at the level I had expected, but any weight loss was exciting. During workouts, we were partners. When he struggled, I was there to provide support and encouragement.

The first crack in the plan came at the beginning of what would be the most draining workout so far. James weighed in prior to starting, and the scale revealed that during the past week he hadn't lost any weight. This was a first since our partnership had begun. I was clearly too slow to wipe the disappointment from my face, because he immediately went into confession mode. He had cheated on the meal plan, he admitted. It was mostly due to a busy work schedule, but there were a few other excuses thrown in for good measure.

I put my poker face back on, encouraged him to stick with the plan, and brushed his challenges off as something that everyone deals with. But I went home that night and confessed frustration to my wife. James had already started seeing results; why had he now jumped off the wagon? More so, James had to lose the weight or face dire consequences. How could he not see it? I was doing my part. The diet wasn't too restrictive. I made certain not to be overly rigid in my plan so that anyone could follow it. Like a good wife, and one who had been through quite a few of these conversations before, Lynn told me to get back up and change my strategy.

Instead of being a workout buddy, I started to approach James with a coachlike mentality. I encouraged him with gentle reminders that this evolution was within his power. We started to make progress again. After a few more weeks the surprising weigh-in truly seemed a blip, and James seemed more committed than ever. That is, until he canceled a workout. I can't remember the reason—just the frustration. We'd been planning to track his weight progress that day, and my guess was that he didn't want to suffer through another confession.

Why did he ask for help if he wouldn't commit for the long haul? Not only was James taking chances with his own life. His decisions would affect his family as well. Moreover, he had lost both of his parents years ago to health problems.

A necessary change was evident, but James seemed to be the only one who didn't see it. It bothered me enough that I asked him about it the next time we met. Instead of admitting his struggles as before, he, too, changed his tactics. He mentioned that some of the habits he'd picked up were "harder to break than you'd think," and that his body "wasn't used to this kind of exercise." The coach in me continued, although James's hesitation and doubt were obvious.

The situation was compounded by our familial relationship. It was one thing for my clients to say that they were struggling—or worse, that they were following meal plans when they really weren't. But I was around James outside of personal training. At family parties I would see him downing multiple sodas, partaking of more than one cheeseburger, and devouring desserts. And I clearly knew how serious his health and weight had become. It was getting uncomfortable for both of us.

I'm sure my wife actually stepped on my foot on more than one occasion as I opened my mouth to speak. I had a hard time watching James sabotage his health. With each get-together it only got worse. Lynn was rightly worried that the next family event might resemble WrestleMania. And yet James still kept coming to workouts. I hadn't lost him yet.

The measures of success, with the exception of a pound being dropped here and there, were much fewer as time went by. A subtle tension started to form between us. I'm sure James could sense my frustration, while I could clearly pick up on his lack of faith in my approach, both short- and long-term. I kept pushing him at our meetings, while afterward venting to my wife about his inability to stop pulling up at the drive-through, and worse, to take such needless chances with his life.

James soon started to make comments about me "not getting it" or just not seeing that "this isn't natural to me." After he canceled three workouts in a row, I changed tactics once again. I picked up the phone and tried to get him to recommit. I even tried to scare him—to make him see that this was about more than losing a few pounds. I emphasized that this lifestyle change could be followed. I was living proof, and my program could get him wherever he wanted to be. I fully believed in the power of the halftime pep talk, but he had to show up—he had to try again. James begrudgingly agreed.

And so now, with "One more try" going through my head, I found myself walking across the gym, trying to gauge how forceful I should be, or if pure apathy should be my last-ditch approach. Before I could get into my personal trainer groove, James stopped me. He was going to try to fight the weight on his own for a bit, he said. He commented about "having the basics" from the instruction I had provided, and thanked me for everything. The reasons flowed from his mouth as if they had been gathering there since the beginning. I lost track of how many excuses he provided before I stopped really listening.

Like a deflated balloon, my bravado sank. I offered generic words of advice, told him to keep in contact if he needed an extra push, and watched him leave the gym. Of course, I couldn't let it go entirely; instead, I went into strategy mode about how I would get through to him at the next family party.

But as I put myself through a rigorous workout to burn off steam from the failed encounter, another thought went through my head. Something was missing. There had to be another way. I pushed a bit harder in my own workout that day, but I couldn't help wondering if I was ever really going to make an impact on someone other than myself.

Dangers of a Black-and-White Worldview

An interesting thing happens when you grow up and have children of your own. A part of you tries to remember all the important lessons you were taught, hoping to impart some of that wisdom to the next generation. Another part of you swears to avoid some of the choices of your parents, happy that you have the power to cure the ills of your own childhood. And a final part embraces the age-old tradition of every generation—that we are smarter, wiser, and more successful than the last.

Part of that arrogance (or, if it's your generation, wisdom) is the knowledge that you have opportunities to change. For my generation, one of those opportunities was gender stereotyping. When I was growing up, it was a societal assumption that I would like cars, dirt, and playing cops and robbers, while my wife was supposed to adore princesses and playing dress-up.

As I grew up on "boy stereotypes," I was surrounded by a black-and-white world. Every time I played a game, we had to choose sides. Sports, cops and robbers, and G-I Joes—all these enforced the idea that there was a good side and a bad side. Maybe we were programmed into these activities because past generations thought that men had the emotional depth of a teacup, and therefore tried to put things in an easy-to-understand format—akin to females of early tribes telling their husbands, "Go. Hunt. Kill animal. Make family happy."

On the opposite end of the spectrum, girl stereotypes ranged into shades of gray. No one won when playing dress-up. There wasn't a wrestling competition between Barbie dolls for control of the pink convertible.

Growing up, while I had three sisters in my life, it was my seven brothers who had the more dominant impact on me. Growing up in a large family, I was constantly in the shadow of what my brothers were accomplishing, usually in team or individual sports. The genesis of my obsession with health, exercise, and fitness grew from there. And as I excelled at sports, one of the traditional boy stereotypes began to take hold: in any game, there was a winner and a loser; there were those who tried harder and those who accepted failure.

As I grew older and more and more obsessed with my own and others' health, this black-and-white worldview only strengthened. I began to understand how much of my own fitness was within my control. I extended that view to others, assuming that those who weren't in shape had voluntarily chosen not to exercise their own control. The world was divided among the motivated and the lazy, the fit and the fat.

True to my boy stereotypes of good vs. bad, I saw the problem as rooted in three main failures (which I'll get to in a minute) of those struggling with their weight. I didn't sit on street corners and scoff at every passerby with a muffin top. It was subtler than that: shaking my head at the line of cars circling a fast-food restaurant, or sighing audibly when an overweight parent at the park was too out of shape to lift his or her child at the playground.

So what were the three failures? First, I was convinced that people used genetics or similar excuses as a crutch. For example, I would hear people at the gym say, "I'm big-boned" or "I was raised to be a meat-and-potatoes kind of guy," literally throwing in the towel. I, on the other hand, was convinced that being healthy was a choice of lifestyle. Being overweight wasn't about how you were raised, or having your family body type working against you. You either wanted to be healthy, or you didn't.

Second, I believed that food and health addictions were also a choice. Habits can be created or broken. After all, I had trained my own body to be addicted to workouts and spinach shakes. If I could do that, you could step away from the french fries, pizza, and ice cream. It frustrated me that people threw their well-being away for a Whopper. It frightened me that for some people a plate of garlic fries or a couple of pints were worth the higher chances of heart disease, stroke, heart attack, and diabetes.

Beyond those stereotypes of failure was a third. It was the one that annoyed me, as a personal trainer, the most. I saw overweight people as taking laziness to the extreme. They tended to have a level of comfort with being overweight. If nothing else, they got used to being sedentary and having an unrestricted diet. The problem had to be compounding itself: they chose to be fat, then they chose to stay fat.

This was one of the reasons that I went into personal training—if they couldn't help themselves, I would do it for them. Unfortunately, I was locked into this mind-set and couldn't see another side. The bigger picture was lost on me, and it would take some tough lessons before I realized I needed a better understanding of those who struggled with weight. How could I help people as a trainer if I didn't understand where they were coming from? If it wasn't as easy as a simple choice, what was it?

My approach worked for me in the sense that it kept me in good shape, encouraged my wife to do the same, and positioned me to raise my two children with the belief that being healthy was a state of mind—one that anyone could control. But this all-or-nothing mentality that sustained me failed to work as a training tool. I simply wasn't having the kind of impact I had hoped for when I started out as a personal trainer. My clients were making progress, but the big lightbulb—the life-changing effect—remained elusive.

My experience with James punctuated this ongoing struggle. Our inability to work together to achieve his goals affected me in a more profound way than any personal training struggles I'd had before. Maybe it was the fact that he was my wife's relative. Maybe I just cared more because I knew him as a person, a friend, and a fellow parent and knew that this was really a matter of life or death.

But as I continued to step away from the experience with James, the moments that stuck with me weren't related to my own missteps at trying to get him to change his lifestyle. Instead, I kept replaying how he had acted, and how an initially successful partnership had devolved into an awkward breakup in the middle of a gym. It was the things he'd said, and perhaps more importantly, everything that he'd left unsaid. For every moment that I told my wife that James didn't get it, I pictured him conveying the same to his wife. And I caught myself multiple times wondering who had it "right" all along.

Suddenly the world wasn't all black and white anymore. I was seeing shades of off-white, charcoal, and everything in between.

And in that more nuanced perspective, a vision developed. I envisioned James and me staring at each other at opposite ends of a long trail on a tall mountain. It was as if I were at the summit, staring down, puzzled by why he couldn't climb up. I had proven that the climb was possible, taken the required steps, and found victory. But for the first time in my life, after having spent so many hours trying to convince others that they could climb the mountain, I switched my perspective. I was the navigator, and I was supposed to guide them around the pitfalls on their path—but did I really know how to traverse the mountain? I had been fit for as long as I could remember—in other words, standing at the summit. If the start of my trail was at the top of the mountain, enjoying the view, how could I understand what it was like for people to find their way from the bottom?

This was the problem: if I couldn't direct from the top, I'd have to go down the mountain myself and prove to everyone just how easy it was to make it all the way back. I found myself in my kitchen thinking about the next steps for my own life, and trying to figure out how I could continue to incorporate fitness into my own activities while helping as many people as I could. If I had learned one lesson from my experience with James, it was that staying the course wasn't going to work. I needed a game-changer.

Bringing My A-Game

If I were to truly understand my clients, and show people how to get and stay fit after being overweight, it was clear that I had to understand myself first. I couldn't rely on any diet book, health magazine, or nutritionist to fill in the blanks and tell me what I was missing. What I missed went far deeper than that. After all, our view of even the tallest mountain depends on where we're standing.

The thought of purposefully getting out of shape flashed briefly in my mind. Then, as the minutes passed, it settled in as if to stay. The thought was a scary one. If you railed against smoking your entire life, how insane would it sound if you turned around and decided to explore the depths of a common chain-smoker?

But there was something powerful, almost intoxicating, about the thought of becoming fat. Individuals who avoid any semblance of being overweight staff the profession of personal training. They view extra pounds as a curse and a weakness. If I could gain weight, and force myself to confront all of my assumptions, the results could only be positive, both for me and for those around me. At the very least, I'd have my time in the sun—I could say that I had experienced what it was like to be overweight, and hopefully reach my audience. At most, I could experience the stereotypical polar opposites that our society deals with on a daily basis. I could be both fat and fit—and hopefully find out what helped and hindered those challenged in finding health.

So, standing in the middle of my kitchen, I decided that this was my best hope to potentially understand weight-loss struggles. I would purposefully gain weight for an entire year, stop exercising, and become a patron at fast-food restaurants across the western United States. After a year, I would turn around and reinvent my own meal plans, workout routines, and general approach to health. In the end, I hoped that I would have a better grasp of what it takes to lose weight and find health.

This was my personal challenge: I would gain the weight, and I would then lose it as quickly as it had packed on. Shockingly (okay, maybe not), Lynn didn't see my idea in the same light. As I explained my grand plans to her that evening, she looked like she was in the latest episode of *Punk'd*. That was the only possible explanation for her husband—the one who made a big deal out of her skipping a workout here and there—"wanting to let himself go."

I was persistent, though. Early in the conversation, she kept bringing up concerns. Her tone was similar to how you'd sound if you tried to logically explain to your child why he couldn't own an elephant for a pet—patient, yet clearly exasperated that any explanation was necessary. But as I continued to push, I could hear her questions and comments change.

Lynn started by wondering if gaining weight for a year was the proper approach, questioning not just the timing but the concept. Then she suggested that a six-month journey to fat, followed by a six-month journey to fit, might be more realistic. And with that shift in perspective, I knew that I had won—and trust me, it's a big deal when the male in a marriage can claim victory.

Over the course of a couple of months, my resolve to pack on the pounds grew, and so did my wife's support. We started to call the journey Fit2Fat2Fit and explored having a website that would chart my progress. We agreed that interested individuals should be able to monitor the physical effects of processed foods and no exercise; and if we could get followers to try to change their health on their own after seeing those effects, all the better.

The approach was simple. I would stop following my meal plans and would instead embrace the typical American diet. In addition, I would cease exercising entirely and would purposefully avoid physical exertion whenever possible (or within, ahem, reason—right, sweetie?).

I would do a weekly weigh-in for the website and would write an ongoing blog, putting into words what it was like to lose the body I had worked so tirelessly to perfect and maintain.

My Favorite Quotes

"Let's change the way we eat,
Let's change the way we live,
Let's change the way we treat each other."
— Tupac

"Even if you're on the right track, you'll get run over if you just sit there."
— Will Rogers

"Nothing tastes as good as healthy feels."
— Unknown

As a fun side project, I'd post a weekly food poll for my followers (if there were any) to vote on. Through the polls, these followers could determine which extreme food challenge I would participate in, assigning an overeating target that I would try to meet. The goal was to show how much my appetite had expanded over time and to entertain the few poor souls who had stumbled upon my website.

I also decided to share my meal plans and workout routines (once I was working the pounds off) with any followers I would have after six months of overindulgence. My goal was to have others join me on the journey back to fit. I wanted us to traverse the mountain together. Knowing that I probably would have lost even my wife's interest, I hoped that someone out there would embrace the sacrifice I was making in the name of research!

As we started to develop the website, my wife brought up one reality I had overlooked—I'd have to tell the parents. If not, they would worry that I had developed a thyroid condition, or that my competitive side had gotten the best of me and I was in some weird competition with my wife (who was pregnant with our second child at the time), wanting to "win" the race to add as many pounds as possible in less than a year.

My Top 10 Food Addictions

- Mountain Dew
- Zingers
- Cinnamon Toast Crunch
- Cap'n Crunch
- Taco Bell Grilled Stuft Burritos
- Peanut butter and Nutella on white bread
- SpaghettiOs
- Hot Pockets
- Chocolate coconut granola bars
- Pringles

If telling my wife was the equivalent of trying to convince a psychiatrist that I wasn't clinically insane, then telling the parents was similar to convincing the surgeon general that his son's lifelong ambition was now to be the Marlboro Man. Both sets (in-laws and my own) spouted off the physical chances I was taking. In what felt like a strange out-of-body experience, they echoed all the rants and speeches I had perfected as a personal trainer.

My dad took a different, perhaps more compelling approach. He asked me the rhetorical question, "What if you never get it back—your old body and your health?" At least I understood where the lack of gray in my life came from! It helped to have my wife on my side, but I could tell as the launch date of Fit2Fat2Fit neared that my closest family and friends, while feigning support, were torn between two views.

On one hand, the idea was like a bad car crash—as much as you wanted to, you couldn't look away. On the other hand, people started giving me reassuring looks that said, "If I had your abs, I'd be insuring them, not abandoning them for a couple doughnuts and french fries."

One of the most important individuals that I needed to tell about my journey, though, was James. After all, I was planning to become what he was. Would he be offended or supportive? I wondered what to expect.

As I explained the plan to him, I tried to highlight that my experience was going to make me a better person and a better personal trainer, giving me insight into something I had never experienced firsthand.

James must have had his own questions about what I was getting myself into, but he was supportive from the outset, and he seemed at least slightly interested in the potential sacrifice I was making. After six months of indulgence, I was going to put myself through the workouts and meal plans he'd experienced, and James would get to be a positive supporter from the sidelines. The roles would be reversed.

But beyond my wife and family, it was most important for those that I had trained before to know why I was starting this trip, and how I hoped that it would help me and others better understand the difficulties and victories around weight loss.

> **I had based my personal training, and so much of my own incessant drive for health, on the certainty that it was easy to be healthy, to make the right choices, and that regardless of your weight, you could always come back. What if I was wrong?**

After months of planning, I eventually found myself ready to depart, eating my last healthy meal before my Fit2Fat2Fit journey officially began.

I thought I would be excited. My wife was—she had been naming all her favorite desserts, which would now be fair game in the house, and her sweet tooth was doing cartwheels in the grocery aisles as our final days of preparation passed. My followers—that is, my family members—were too; they had already chosen my first food challenge of 12 Krispy Kreme doughnuts.

While I felt a measure of their anticipation, I was dealing with some other emotions. First and foremost, I was scared. Sure, I was already afraid that I'd become the "guy who vomits while stuffing his face with doughnuts" on YouTube, but I was scared mostly of the uncertainty. I had based my personal training, and so much of my own incessant drive for health, on the certainty that it was easy to be healthy, to make the right choices, and that regardless of your weight, you could always come back. What if I was wrong?

Soon my self-doubt was taking over. What if I really did have to struggle to get the weight off? Mere hours from diving into the 12 doughnuts now adorning my kitchen table, I started to wonder how much I had bet on a single hand of blackjack. In addition to my waistline, I pondered what the effect would be on my marriage, children, job, and relationships. It seemed like an awful chance to take for an unrestricted diet and a few "aha" moments about what it's like to be overweight.

Fully supportive, my wife never asked me if I wanted to back out, but if she had, I wonder what my honest answer would have been. As I stewed about what I was undertaking, mostly I thought of James and others like him—I pictured them sitting at the bottom of that mountain, staring up at what seemed impossible. They needed someone who understood. And with that, I grabbed my plate of doughnuts and asked my wife to hit the play button for my first video of Fit2Fat2Fit. Let the games begin.

A Closet Full of Clothes, with Nothing to Wear

Just two months later, I was standing in front of my closet staring at my clothes and having the thought that every woman has probably dealt with: I had a closet full of clothes, with nothing to wear.

My conundrum, however, wasn't due to being out of fashion. It was due to trying to find an outfit to wear to work that didn't accentuate the gut I was now steadily developing. As a fit individual, I had tended to gravitate to form-fitting clothes. Now, that adjective no longer had the same connotations.

Everything I tried on shouted, "Yes, I'm gaining weight at an inordinate pace!" And to make matters worse, as far as I knew I didn't have more than a smattering of followers outside my core family and friends who knew that I was doing this on purpose.

When I was fit, any self-confidence issues I had consisted of thinking I could lose a little on my love handles, an obsession that would always earn a well-placed eye roll from my wife. Now, a little voice in my head craved to know what those around me were thinking. Even worse, I now believed that every person who knew me before the journey was thinking one of two things: 1) What has he done to himself? 2) Did he just now discover cookies?

The critical problem was that I cared how others perceived me. I desperately wanted to talk to strangers and acquaintances alike about my journey. In truth, any struggles with self-esteem when I was fit were internal. While I had the worst inner critic, there was still only one of me. Now, as I started to gain weight, my self-esteem issues became an obsession. I feared that everyone noticed every new pound—yes, even strangers.

To avoid that problem, I wished that I could stay home, but my weight gain was equally shocking to my wife. She would catch a view of me in a tight shirt or more scantily clad and teasingly poke fun at my "cottage cheese" butt or my quickly deteriorating posture. Instead of laughing and moving on, I took such comments personally. I'd check the mirror, watching for any cottage cheese resemblance. I'd wear the least-form-fitting clothes I had, because it was easier to hide what was happening than to embrace it.

Paradoxically, even as I was using clothes to hide my weight, I used words to expose it. I'd visit with friends (even ones who knew about the journey), and before they could ask me how I was, I would make comments like, "Can you believe how much I've changed?" I found it was easier to point out the obvious and get them to talk about their "judgment" of me, than to sit back and wonder what was going through their heads.

What disturbed me most, however, was that a key stereotype already seemed to be in question. If I was suddenly feeling the pressure of wondering what those around me were thinking, what did people who had struggled with this their entire lives feel? If I, the personal trainer, felt hesitant to leave the house, what were the Jameses of the world feeling? And how did those feelings impact their ability to stay focused on their goals?

As I grabbed the closest thing to a non-form-fitting shirt I could find and got ready for work at my med-tech job (I'd put most of my training clients on hold while I undertook Fit2Fat2Fit), I realized that this journey wasn't about gaining pounds and reporting back on my blog. There was an emotional and mental component that I hadn't anticipated. This was going to be much more difficult than I had imagined.

As I eased my growing midsection behind the steering wheel, started my car, and headed to work, one thought hit me. The games had indeed begun. And I wasn't anywhere close to winning.

CHAPTER 3

NO ONE SAID IT WOULD BE EASY

We are all creatures of habit. Regardless of what goes on in our lives, it seems like we're constantly searching for organization and structure. When I was fit, my routine could best be described as militant. I ate certain foods at certain times, prepared certain ways. There was a streak of obsessive-compulsive disorder (OCD) in my daily routine—something Lynn would constantly poke fun at, trying to throw me off my game by moving food around in the cupboards and refrigerator and (allegedly!) scheduling family and friend activities that caused me to adjust my schedule.

To be fair to my wife, I can't imagine that it was enjoyable for her to wait, on our rare date nights, so that I could get my workout in first. Or to have me using the blender as an alarm clock as I made my morning spinach shake while the rest of our family was still in a deep slumber. Let's just say that when romantic partners across the country are waking their other half up while the children sleep, these significant others are hoping it's not for a green smoothie!

It's funny what they say about routines being all about habit. With more pounds added to my hips than I cared to admit, my old routine was nowhere to be found. But like many of us, I didn't take long to find another, less fun one.

This Tuesday morning was different, though. I rolled out of bed and fell right into my new routine. I stumbled my way into the shower. I reached for my razor, setting it back down once I realized that I'd put my "manscaping" (the tried-and-true tradition of removing that "manly" body hair in order to become more . . . manly) on hold. It wasn't hard to remember, given that Lynn had started asking for late-night escapades "with the lights off, please!"

I picked out some clothes that hid my bulging belly and ever-expanding bottom and tried to drown my disgust with my physical appearance in a bowl of one of my newly established addictions—Cinnamon Toast Crunch. After finishing off the box, I checked my e-mail, cleared out the spam that claimed it could help me "lose 10 pounds overnight," and left the house to make the long drive from Utah to Idaho, a drive I made three times a week for my "day job."

I did my best to mask my new routine by "mixing it up"—instead of McDonald's, I'd treat myself to Taco Bell or Burger King. I would eat the fast food of the day, realizing with every bite that the initial guilt of caloric intake had been replaced by an unnatural craving for anything fried in oil and grease.

Getting home after another long drive back, I would make two meals: a healthy option for my wife and kids, and the "typical American cuisine" (such as SpaghettiOs) for me. After I'd finished my gourmet dinner that particular Tuesday night, I logged in to clear out a new bunch of spam e-mail, convinced that the only people actively following my blog were my wife and my parents.

A Greater Purpose

That's when I got Megan's e-mail. And my world changed.

Megan was in her early 40s, she wrote, living in Florida. Currently, she was of average height and weighed over 240 pounds. She wanted to tell me her story, she said, and I hung on every word. Megan hadn't been overweight her entire life. She'd been in reasonable shape for most of it, actually. But life got in the way: divorce, dating, difficult relationships, a second marriage, moving cross-country and back, and a stressful job added pounds along with gray hairs.

Before the additional stress, Megan had been a runner and had enjoyed yoga. She'd embraced her laps at the local pool and had even dabbled in weight lifting. In those days Megan had loved her body—every single curve. Yet with extra stress and extra weight, she noticed changes in her personality as well as her shape, and she didn't like either. Once an extrovert, she turned into an introvert who exercised less, ate more junk food, and spent larger parts of her time depressed.

Megan didn't give up, though. She'd start exercising, find some incremental success, and start to feel better—but the improvement never lasted during a big life upheaval. The longest she had stayed the course had been about three months, resulting in weight loss of over 24 pounds. Then her mother passed away, and soon every lost pound found its way back onto Megan's body.

What struck me most about Megan's story came next. She was tired of being overweight, tired of trying and failing. She put into words some of the desires her weight had stopped her from experiencing. Megan wanted nothing more than to be healthy and active. She wanted to find a routine and stick to it. She wanted to wear high heels again, and return to the social experiences she had robbed herself of as life got more and more complicated.

Everything she saw as wrong with her life came back to the weight. Megan's health, daily routine, and attitude were dominated by her lack of ability to reach her fitness goals. On a daily basis she was presented with various ways to lose weight, including familial pressure from her sister to join Weight Watchers. But she stayed away, wanting to avoid the pressure exerted by her family, and mostly afraid of failing in front of others.

After countless blog posts, food challenges, and weigh-in videos on my part, and spam e-mails on the part of the world, someone had reached out to me with heartfelt words I hadn't expected. In addition to sharing her story, Megan also thanked me. She had committed to being a follower of my journey, she told me, because she, too, wanted to achieve her goal. My journey had resonated with her. Maybe it was the forum (an anonymous blog was easier to follow in the comfort of her own living room, after all); maybe it was the approach. Whatever it was, she found in me a silent partner with whom to advance her own health goals.

I reread Megan's e-mail two or three times. With every word, I felt my own sense of apathy starting to splinter. A new emotion was creeping through: even if my routine didn't allow for much energy these days, I felt hopeful suddenly—and it was revitalizing.

Suck It Up

When you find out you're going to be a father, everyone tells you that there are no roadmaps. I remember all the talk around me about the sense of discovery, the wonder of experiences you never thought you'd have, and the inescapable terror you feel each day because you're no longer sure that you're doing things right. My conclusion, as I heard these warnings, was that preparation for fatherhood would be a waste of time. It would be better to figure it out as I went along.

My wife, on the other hand, sent me to the local bookstore to buy scads of books about what to do before, during, after, and while you're bringing a tiny human being into the world. As the big day got closer, she became even more prepared. True to form, she read the books from cover to cover, and she proceeded to nest the entire house in anticipation.

Meanwhile, I stayed committed to my nonpreparation. I figured that parenthood would simply work itself out. I might need a few pointers on how to properly change a diaper or give fatherly advice farther down the line, but I was sure I'd know instinctively how to help during childbirth. I would be a natural parent. I'd care for my children and teach them the finer points of the Cover 2 scheme in football. And I just knew I'd deliver the perfect dating speech to my son or daughter when the teenage years struck.

Then our first child arrived, and I wished I'd been the one reading the books. As I held my precious baby in my arms, winging it didn't seem like the best strategy after all.

It shouldn't come as a shock, then, that I approached gaining what I thought would be 50 to 60 pounds in much the same way. I didn't spend an inordinate amount of time researching the medical, physical, emotional, and mental challenges that were before me.

My Top Five Anti-Workouts of Fit2Fat

- Vegging out during football Saturdays and Sundays and Mondays, and sometimes Thursdays
- Reaching into my pocket to pay the neighborhood kid $10 to mow my lawn because I am too tired
- Watching a movie with my daughter Kale'a instead of playing with her
- Volunteering to go grocery shopping instead of cleaning the house
- Making date night a movie-in night because I am too miserable to go out after a food challenge

I'd convinced myself that the first half of my journey was purely physical. Like dating, marriage, and parenting, however, becoming fat walloped me upside the head—and I wasn't prepared for any of it.

The physical side of becoming overweight goes well beyond, say, the sheer amount of trans fat you consume or the pounds you gain. The bodily effects are enormous: added weight gives equal favor to expanding waist, hips, and bottom, all growing proportionally (or in the case of my bottom, not so proportionally). For guys, you even need to deal with unexpected man boobs!

As the pounds did their job, I began to realize that my body was not only expanding, but moving more slowly. On top of that, I had been introduced to chafing. Honestly, though, I was more afraid of potential stretch marks than I was of chafed skin, so I would put Lynn through the horrible experience of "rubbing the Buddha" with her pregnancy stretch-mark cream.

As the months went by, the chafing appeared more frequently. My man boobs, once the subject of a self-deprecating anecdote on my weekly blog, gathered copious amounts of sweat when I did something as innocuous as taking out the garbage, and the sides of my pectoral region began to feel inflamed.

Worse was the act of walking. My wife probably thought I was getting too lazy to even hand her the drink sitting on the table before me, and she was right: I dreaded physical movement of any kind, but especially genuine exertion.

One thing was painfully clear. If I, as a budding fat person, was already dreading a walk up the stairs, how did my overweight clients feel when I ruthlessly subjected them to 25 push-ups and an equal number of sit-ups in front of unsupportive onlookers at the gym?

As the growing feeling of exhaustion exacerbated the chafing and physical pain, I lost my will to contribute at home. Prior to gaining weight, I was an overachiever in the household. I did most of the cooking (to make sure I was "eating healthy"—but it earned me brownie points with my wife despite that selfish motivation) and tried to be as helpful as I could with my family.

With every added pound, both the effort and the desire to be helpful slipped away. Scarier, the guilt I initially felt at putting the household upkeep on Lynn seeped away too. I'm ashamed to admit that I was comfortable lying on the couch while she balanced housework, children, and dinner preparation after her own long day at work.

Early on, when she asked me to help out, I would begrudgingly agree, although she'll tell you I complained about it with much more vigor than I put into the actual activity. But as time passed, and I gained more weight, Lynn moved from open frustration to quiet resignation. I knew which was worse.

I sat on the couch, too tired to play with my two-year-old girl, too hesitant to invite an extra bout of chafing in my oversized body. And once I'd moved from the living room to the bedroom each evening, fluffing my pillow was about the extent of what I could do in bed.

If my home life provided countless reminders of how physically unprepared I was for going from Fit2Fat, my work life supplemented the emotional and mental evidence of the same. And in a medical workplace, the reminders and evidence never leave you.

In my line of work as a neuromonitoring tech, scrubs are a daily requirement. On some days, the usual cloth scrubs aren't available. When I was fit, the occasional need for paper scrubs never caused problems. As I gained weight, however, paper scrubs became problematic, both for chafing and durability. I knew I had gained more weight than I had expected to when the XL scrubs were uncomfortably tight.

As I set up in the operating room one day, bending over to adjust some settings, I heard a gigantic rip: my large bottom had caused my pants to rip in half. I glanced down at the flimsy remains and was horrified—and grateful that I had not gone commando that day!

Worse still, my workday had only begun. I perfected the art of using one hand to hold my pants together while doing my assigned tasks to get through the rest of the surgery. I couldn't help but laugh at myself for my predicament. This was exactly the type of thing I had imagined would happen—almost comical experiences in which my body had clearly outgrown what I was used to. It was like being a teenager again: awkward.

I had approached gaining weight with the thought that any strain would be related to embarrassing situations like this. I had visions of dribbling food down my front, or trying to wear T-shirts so small that they resembled midriff tops and I looked like a drag queen.

And yet—despite my anticipation of such events—my embarrassment over them was palpable, extending far beyond the hospital doors.

I sensed societal judgment wherever I went. If I ordered a large meal at a restaurant, I could see the server looking me up and down (and not in a "How you doin'?" sort of way). There was a look of exasperation when a fellow airline passenger realized that I'd be sitting next to him or her. And when family and friends saw me huddled on the couch and out of breath, even my closest supporters shook their heads or rolled their eyes.

It helped a bit that I had expected the embarrassment part. As hurt as some of the judgments made me feel, I wasn't surprised that my physical changes would elicit reactions, whether teasing or serious, and I felt that I could let any hurt feelings roll off my stretch-marked back. What I *hadn't* expected was the fear.

Back at work that day, as I sheepishly made my way to the pile of XXL scrubs ("graduating" from XL), I heard a commotion down the hall. As I exited the room, I could see that one of the other people working in the hospital was in distress not far away. Someone like me, I thought, though I didn't know him well. This person, who was severely overweight, had collapsed just outside the front door. I found myself selfishly thinking that this could have been me.

Staff members rushed around, trying to aid the man, who had apparently suffered a major heart attack. It was so bad that the crew helping out had to revive him. I wasn't a part of the efforts to save him, but the impact of this event was greater than I'd ever expected.

The medical implications of my weight gain had been Mom's greatest worry when I first opened up to her about my plan. And on a weekly basis, I would be inundated with questions, not only from her but from friends, the doctors and nurses I worked with, and even strangers, about the danger to my heart, liver, and kidneys, and potential risk for diabetes. Most people asked me about the extra stress on my body and voiced their concerns loud and clear.

I always thought I would be fine, especially at the outset. It was only for six months, after all. When my wife would mention health concerns, I'd tell her that by the time my body was truly at risk, I'd already be losing the weight as quickly as I'd gained it.

But that was before the incident at the hospital. I had no doubt that my coworker's heart attack was directly tied to the excess weight he was carrying. Indeed, with my concern about ripped scrubs, I had been living in the shallow end of the pool. And I was in denial.

From that point on, with every weigh-in, the vision of small shirts and ripped scrubs was replaced by the thought of the very real danger I was putting my body through. This wasn't just a cute blog story for strangers to follow.

I'd spent most of my adult life trying to convince family, friends, and clients that they were playing Russian roulette with their health. And now it was my turn to play. Experiencing the game was a much more difficult task than I'd realized.

And with every cheeseburger or lazy day on the couch, I was getting farther and farther removed from myself emotionally. I was tense. I lost my patience easily. I wasn't happy anymore.

Megan's e-mail opened my eyes, allowing me to see past my own fears, and helped me remember the reason I'd started this project in the first place. Besides, I was already accomplishing one of my chief goals—to inspire as many people as possible to improve their health, and to help them by being honest with and about myself.

Be Careful What You Blog For

I hadn't realized that anyone was paying attention to my experiment beyond the small number of followers I had developed. My hope for the website was to attract people through personal relationships as the journey progressed—family would tell friends, friends would tell friends, and at the end of the ordeal, I could get through to a far greater audience than I would by reaching two or three individual clients in the gym.

There had been some interest close to home. My local newspaper had written an article, one of the more popular local radio stations had conducted an interview on air, and a local TV news station had run a five-minute story early in one of their evening broadcasts. As more publicity hit, I noticed that my in-box was filling with more than spam.

I enjoyed reading and carefully responding to each of my messages. In every Facebook response I sent, I tried to answer a question or thank a follower for taking the time to send a message. The e-mails I received carried me through my depressed days, giving me extra patience with my family and myself.

And then one day I got a wholly different e-mail. Having participated in an interview that I thought would appear on a lightly traveled fitness website, I was informed that the interview and article would actually appear . . . on the front page of Yahoo.com, the very next day!

The next morning I checked Yahoo.com every 30 minutes or so, eager to see the piece. Every time I looked I was greeted by gossip about Demi Moore and Jennifer Aniston. When the article finally did hit, my telephone began ringing—radio stations, television shows, and family and friends called in rapid succession. Once again I wasn't prepared, though in this case I'll give myself a break. I'm not sure that anyone could have prepared for the avalanche of interest that followed. In fact, the volume of hits crashed my website, and I frantically tried to figure out how to get my story back online.

With no pun intended, this attention was difficult to digest. Before I knew it, I was spending my time on three major activities—being interviewed, reading/responding to e-mails, and eating (hey, I still had a routine to maintain!). I suddenly had a platform from which to make an impact far greater than I had ever dared to imagine.

At the peak of my weight gain, I sat in one of the prep rooms of *The Dr. Oz Show*, trying to comprehend this whirlwind. We had walked through what the interview would entail—I'd have the opportunity to tell the world what was so great about my own spinach shake recipe from the fit days, and Dr. Oz would educate his audience on the medical impact that an unrestricted diet and lack of exercise could truly have.

I was just over a week away from the end of Fit2Fat and the beginning of Fat2Fit. Almost ready to start back on the journey to fitness, I was already making preparations to get as many followers as possible on board to lose the weight with me.

But *The Dr. Oz Show* provided more than another avenue to reach potential followers. It was a collision of the two realities of my journey so far:

As America's favorite doc explained the differences between a healthy and unhealthy kidney and liver, I got chills of unease. My wife had the same reaction. Perhaps her worry was even greater since it had begun earlier in the journey. We had started to track my blood pressure, and she knew just how high it had gotten.

On the flip side, the amount of support I received after the Yahoo.com interview was incredible. I was always behind on e-mails, had countless interviews lined up before me, and hadn't seen my children in a week. All in the name of trying to reach a greater audience—to wake them up to what typical Americans were doing to themselves. For every fearful moment, every shred of doubt, there was an encouraging e-mail. Some followers poured their own fears and frustrations into e-mails, hoping that someone would give *them* support.

Top Three Guilty Pleasures

- Waking up in the middle of the night starving and eating a bowl of cereal or a whole can of Pringles
- Stopping by the gas station to pick up Zingers and an energy drink on my way to work
- Quitting manscaping, leaving me more time to do other things, like eat

Even personal trainers were weighing in on the matter, startled that I would take the steps I had to understand my clientele, but appreciative of their own changing understanding of what it meant to have so much weight to lose.

In my fit days, the routine had been control and order. Then, as my journey evolved, I became uncontrolled and reckless. These days, I needed to understand the true dangers and consequences of an unhealthy lifestyle, while supporting a growing network of followers who were looking for a path to their own health.

While I may have been unprepared in many ways for my experience with becoming overweight, I had an almost endless list of expectations going into it. But here's the thing about expectations and plans: they don't account for life. Nothing ever happens as you expect it to. There are challenges that you aren't sure you're equipped to deal with, that you're not ready for. And your life becomes so much more complicated than it used to be.

As I mentioned earlier, I always thought that people chose to be healthy or not. But I learned that it's not as simple as "deciding" to be healthy on any particular day, especially when you haven't been before. You need good reasons, strong will, internal motivation, and community support to change your life for the better.

The irony is that I had to do the opposite of my followers to change my own life around. I needed good reasons, strong will, internal motivation, and above all community support during the months of weight gain. But the result was the same—as my body changed on the outside and within, my life changed for the better.

It was no longer about me. Fit2Fat2Fit had become about a group of individuals deciding that we were going to transform our lives. My idea for the journey may have been the catalyst, but now every one of us was in this together. Putting health first was a community effort, and I knew that we all needed each other to succeed.

Yes, I now know what it's like to be physically overweight. I learned how to deal with snoring, chafing, and extreme exhaustion. I ripped a few scrubs in the process. But as I noted earlier, being overweight is so much more than a physical experience. There is an emotional toll.

The enormity of self-doubt you inherit isn't something that can be described. The fear of life-threatening effects on your health becomes all too real. And the sense of isolation—from your community, as well as society as a whole—never leaves you. But I finally knew what it felt like, and that is the wisdom I had sought.

Amidst the turmoil of my life, though, and amidst my feelings of isolation, was a greater realization that people are never as alone as they think they are. My followers, especially Megan, had made me realize that every "Like" on Facebook or comment on a blog post was coming from someone who could be struggling with weight, looking for guidance and inspiration, or longing to connect.

But with thousands of e-mails pouring in daily, the responsibility had started to sink in. I hoped my weekly updates, posts, and tweets would reach people in a way that truly helped them. The irony wasn't lost on my wife, nor on me. Months back, alone in my kitchen, reflecting on the failed personal training experience with James, I had been frustrated by the lack of impact I was making. Success wasn't a guarantee—either before my journey or now.

As I reached six months, the fear for my health and the unknowns about whether I would take the weight off still occupied my thoughts daily. The goal, after all, was to help people reach their goals with me. But it was no longer about me. Fit2Fat2Fit had become about a group of individuals deciding that we were going to transform our lives. My idea for the journey may have been the catalyst, but now every one of us was in this together.

Putting health first was a community effort, and I knew that we all needed each other to succeed.

CHAPTER 4

THE ICK FACTOR: A WIFE'S PERSPECTIVE

When I was younger, dating a host of eligible bachelors, I'd always see if each new person could pass my simple first-date test—you know, the one where you see if you can make it through a meal with enough to talk about before you turn to engaging conversation subjects like, "Wow, this water seems fresh!"

And while it may be true that no first date leads to a second date without "common interests," that need for commonality seems to become less important the longer a relationship lasts. By the time you're staring at the possibility of marriage, the joining of your differences is what starts to create a lifelong bond.

At least that's what I tell myself when I look at the vast differences between my husband and me. If it's not painfully obvious by now, my husband loves being fit. It actually defines him. From the moment we started dating, I was introduced to a world of maximum exercise, minimal unhealthy food, and clear rules around anything considered a treat.

I, on the other hand, am a foodie. I live to eat. You can toss away fancy jewelry, flowers, and a carriage ride in the snow. Give me a four-course meal at my favorite restaurant, and the deal is sealed.

I'm not a natural exerciser. I've dabbled in running, but physical activity has never been at the top of my to-do list. Exercising has always been a fun diversion, nothing less and nothing more.

And my biggest weakness is dessert. Cookies, cakes, and pies were welcome guests in my home in the pre-Drew days—not as the occasional treat, but every day.

That's how I decided that opposites attract, at least for us. How else could you explain a fitness freak marrying a food lover? In many ways Drew was there to improve my health, filling our house with the right foods and encouraging me to exercise.

As for my part, I got Drew out of the house for romantic dates and dinners with friends, teaching him that it was all right to take the day off once in a while, and even more okay to order a dessert . . . or two. That was the balance we found in our life and our marriage.

Drew's worldview dominated the weekdays, as we made daily spinach shakes and prepared meals for the week as if we were preparing for a natural disaster. The weekends lent themselves to my exploits as we relaxed our supernatural standards.

Needless to say, I lived for date nights. I loved the whole process—dressing up just a bit more, eating better food, and getting out of the house for an evening. Once we had children, it became even more important to act like adults and enjoy our time together.

To say that Fit2Fat2Fit changed the balance in our marriage would be the understatement of the century. Although I was completely supportive as the journey got under way, our marriage evolved greatly as Drew added pounds, and by the end of the Fit2Fat stage, we were the perfect image of imbalance.

Nothing illustrates the change more than date night. The transition was subtle at first. We'd go out, and instead of Drew scouring the menu to find the healthiest thing he could, he'd let flavor dictate his choice. I noticed a pleasant change of pace: for the first time during our marriage, we were allowed to order like foodies.

That enjoyable phase didn't last long. With two children, our jobs, and Drew's journey eating up more and more of our time, date night took on a different role. Drew was now totally invested in his weekly food challenges, trying to prove just how much his tastes and appetite had evolved. As a result, our alone time was replaced by a quick meal for me so that I could hold the video camera while he tried to really pig out (or eat a real pig).

Soon enough, however, date night didn't even get us out of the house. There was no more need to dress up; my inner foodie remained where she was—inside. Drew's new eating habits had changed something in me. I suddenly took on the role of the healthy eater, because I was tired of seeing his typical American cuisine on our kitchen counter every single night.

The tipping point came one evening after the kids had gone to bed. I was looking forward to some quiet time and relaxation. But Drew had other ideas. I found him sitting on the couch, complaining about his stomach and how full he was from the week's food challenge. And then I noticed the bottle in his hands.

Sheepishly, he asked for my help. Would I mind rubbing some stretch-mark lotion on his belly? He was just too tired to do it himself, he said. In that moment, the thought, *How much do I love him?* flashed through my mind.

I grabbed the bottle and started rubbing lotion over his big, hairy belly.

It was in that moment that I saw the real changes in Drew . . . and the changes in us.

As Drew was gaining weight, another voluntary physical change took place: he stopped shaving his chest and arms. Body hair had always been something Drew abhorred. There seemed to be a correlation between his gym obsessions and what he called "manscaping." The more fit he was, the more razors there were in our bathroom.

Sixty pounds later, in a conversation I had with one of my closest friends, I was able to put into words the difficulties that this journey had brought—physically, at least.

A true foodie compares the world and life experiences to food. So when my friend asked me what it was like to have an overweight husband, when I had been accustomed to his flat stomach, food, of all things, came to mind.

I've dated men of all shapes and sizes. Some were skinny, some heavy. And others were fit. I didn't care. Body weight is a little like salmon. No matter whether it's smoked, raw, or grilled, salmon is delightful. More often than not, I've enjoyed a little "salmon" in my life.

I've also dated men of various "manscapes." Drew represented one end of the spectrum; his body was a well-manicured wonderland. But since I didn't mind body hair, I certainly never demanded that Drew shave. Body hair is a little like peanut butter. It's great in the right place and quantity.

The problem, then, wasn't the weight or the hair; it was the combination. Drew gained an immense amount of weight and let an extraordinary amount of body hair grow. While each of these "additions" was individually palatable, together they resulted in . . . peanut butter–smeared salmon. And trust me: salmon never goes well with peanut butter.

This unusual and off-putting combination caused some awkward moments in our marriage, and specifically in our sex life.

Fitting sex into a marriage with a two-year-old and a newborn is hard in itself. You need to choose your "moments" wisely, because they're vital to staying sane through the rigors of work, kids, and life in general. Given that peanut butter–coated salmon was our plat du jour—it was that or nothing—I started compensating in the bedroom. First, it was a simple adjustment. Our bedroom light had a dimmer that I started to use. To this day, I'm unsure whether Drew noticed any difference back then (he is a man, after all), but it helped me.

Yet the dimmed lights could do only so much. Drew's feelings were probably hurt when I asked for the lights to actually be off, but since I needed the adjustment, he adjusted.

Like many young families, we have various night-lights scattered through our house. We pretend that it's for the kids, to keep them from getting scared in the dark. In reality, it's to help overtired parents avoid tripping over toys, pacifiers, and baby clothes and falling down the stairs.

One evening, Drew and I came to the realization that the physical attraction and connection that had been so strong for us had somehow splintered through this journey. That night, after he had turned off the lights and climbed into bed, I had gently asked him to turn off the night-light, too. That's when I realized that my "close my eyes and think of England" approach to our current sex life wasn't working miracles for our relationship. The spark was barely burning anymore.

Despite my comparison to salmon and peanut butter, to say that this change in our relationship was due only to some added weight and body hair would be unfair to both Drew and me. Yes, he looked different—but the physical changes caused emotional changes in my husband. And *they* made the superficial adjustments hard to bear.

My husband has always been a humble person. The old Drew never flaunted his body or his fitness, even to me. He was more critical of the further "work" he needed to put into his body than he was complimentary of the results he had earned. The new Drew's self-esteem had completely disappeared, taking "humble" to unplumbed depths. It was as if his waistline and confidence were on the same sliding scale.

At first it was bearable, even cute. Drew had started to ask the question I considered reserved for girlfriends and wives looking for some male support: "Does this make me look fat?"

But questions turned to complaints. And the complaining evolved into whining. Some days, I felt like I had three children living in the household. Trying to keep my husband's self-worth above water was now a full-time job. And with the initial lack of followers on his blog discouraging him, my attempts to help him feel better about himself seemed less and less effective.

Drew carried himself more heavily these days. Back in the day, when I dated men who were heavier, or those who hadn't heard of manscaping, they had been comfortable with how their bodies looked. Their weight didn't bring them down.

In contrast, Drew's weight brought both of us down. I loved my husband as much as I ever had, but I wasn't nearly as attracted to him as before. Drew didn't believe in himself anymore, and I was struggling to believe enough for both of us.

When Drew first changed his diet and exercise habits, I believed that we were in for a glorious six months. I was going to party openly and enthusiastically, no longer needing to sneak desserts into the house on a weekly basis.

Maybe it was the fact that my desserts started disappearing before I had a chance to eat a bite. Perhaps the sight of my once-fit husband sporting a gut that would make Santa Claus jealous affected me more than I'd expected. For whatever reason, we started to switch roles. Not only was I backing away from the foodie in me, but I started working out regularly!

The more Drew damaged his body, the more self-conscious I was about what I was doing for mine. I started following his old meal plans, and even pushed myself to compete in local races. I tried to understand what the changes in our marriage had triggered within me.

I wondered if balance was necessary in any relationship, especially as it relates to finding long-lasting health. Our old system had worked, I concluded, because two approaches helped create that delicate equilibrium. Every time I would get a little out of control, Drew would pull me back. And every time he resembled a military general, I turned on my date-night charm.

With the roles reversed, our marriage was now completely out of whack, and I found myself in the role of obsessive health nut. While I couldn't force Drew to eat better, I could ensure that my children and I ate responsibly and got enough exercise.

Is this why so many people fail when battling against being overweight? Perhaps they lack a counterbalance to pull them back on track when things get rough.

It's possible that this is the cause of many personal trainers' inability to understand what it's like to be overweight. They aren't surrounded by the same temptations, and don't understand what it's like to be comfortably sedentary.

My birthday is three days removed from that of our two-year-old.

Our joint party was held at a local activity center. We had upwards of 25 people on the way, and the amount of coordination for what seemed like a simple party was absolutely overwhelming. The day started out simply—getting the kids ready to go, making sure that we had our reservation, the cake, presents, and plans.

Trying to coordinate multiple children in a crowded place comes with challenges. Even as you're hosting, you don't want to miss a minute of your child's day.

In the joint birthday world, you're also opening presents yourself, thanking everyone for taking time out of their day, and trying to enjoy yourself. And at this activity center, I was also on point for teaching my daughter how to roller-skate, helping her up after face-plants in the bounce house, and teaching her some skills in the arcade.

Drew, on the other hand, got winded easily and thus chose to avoid the various activities available. In fact, every time I looked over at Drew, I saw him eating. I didn't know whether to be annoyed or jealous.

I woke up the next day feeling like I hadn't slept at all. Standing in the kitchen, attempting to get the household moving for the day, I tried to explain my exhaustion to my husband. His answer was what had recently become the norm—a competition to show who was the more exhausted/tired/overworked one. Drew complained that he hadn't slept either and that just walking up the stairs made him tired, let alone keeping the party together the day before.

This triggered my meltdown. It had probably been coming for months. Drew and I had fought more in these last six months than we had in our entire six-year marriage. But at some point, everyone reaches a limit.

I told my husband that if I didn't keep reminding myself this journey was temporary, I'd be having serious thoughts about getting a divorce attorney. Yes, it was just a marital fight, but I was ranting at a person I didn't recognize, let alone like very much. This fight, our low point, cast a harsh light on the true effects this journey was having on our marriage.

Men are simple creatures; they're convinced that the key to being "desirable" is to be fit, handsome, or romantic. This is ironic to me. Particularly once you're married, isn't the physical attraction kind of a given?

What married women will tell you—their unwritten secret—is that there's nothing sexier than a man doing the dishes. And this is what was so attractive and endearing about the old Drew. He was always willing to go the extra mile, and not just on the treadmill. He claimed his share of "night shifts" with the kids and helped around the house every day.

This is what I said to everyone who asked me whether I was still attracted to my husband, without his washboard stomach. In truth, I would have preferred an actual washboard. Who was this man without self-esteem who seemed content to have the world revolve around his journey? And what had he done with my helpful and willing husband?

And while it was easy to feel fearful when doctors or friends mentioned the potential harm Drew was doing to his body, I was more scared of the impact on our marriage.

Later, I came to a realization, both about the journey and about my husband. In the end, Drew wasn't a different person at all. It's not like a few doughnuts had caused him to care less about our household, our children, or me. He simply *couldn't* translate his caring into action.

The effect of added weight goes well beyond needing marital reassurance or extra-large sweat pants. Weight gain changes a person's desire to do the things many take for granted, like playing with their kids, getting off the couch, or being motivated to help out around the house. There's a barrier that's not easy to see when you're healthy and fit—a physical and emotional barrier, the combination of which can stop even those with the best intentions from thriving.

Fit2Fat2Fit seemed like such an innocent idea when first proposed. I liked the thought that my husband could reach an audience so much greater than he could as a personal trainer. And I loved the fact that he decided to take a journey that would provide him deeper insight into himself and the most important aspects of his life.

But I was naive in thinking that the avenue to that goal would be a few extra pounds. Just six months later, my date nights were mundane, and I found that I was dealing with more fights and turmoil than I'd bargained for.

This was not just about the cost of a radical lifestyle change anymore. Being overweight is never a purely personal issue. It's not a struggle that one self-contains. It affects everyone, in one way or another.

I waited with longing for the old Drew to come back.

PART TWO

FAT2FIT

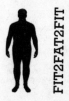

CHAPTER 5

COLD TURKEY

The reality of the situation had started to hit me the night before, but only now, peering into the garbage can, did I realize what I had just given up.

Don't get me wrong. I was excited—I had started dreaming of this phase. I dreamed about how good it would feel to get back to my healthy lifestyle, back to "me."

Last night's activities had been Lynn's idea. She thought that it would be cathartic to have an official event where I went through the pantry, refrigerator, and various hiding places to get rid of the processed and unhealthy foods that had accumulated in our house.

Some things were easy to part with: I was quite sure that I wouldn't miss the SpaghettiOs or the little piles of "meatballs" hidden at the bottom of the can. And while they had been tasty, I could do without the peanut butter sandwiches (on white bread) and energy drinks that had accompanied me during lengthy car rides to and from work.

But I was having a hard time letting two items go. What would I be without my daily bowls of Cinnamon Toast Crunch? How could I function without my liter of Mountain Dew? And why did I let myself get to the point where I was going to miss these food items as if they were my third and fourth children?

Yet under the watchful eye of my wife, that's what I did. It was the loss of those two items that brought me to stare longingly into the garbage can on a freezing November morning. Clearly the catharsis of my wife's plan the previous evening hadn't been as effective as we had hoped it would be.

This day was also a celebration, I reminded myself as I closed the lid of the garbage can. I was going to get back to taking care of my body and treating it right. It was time to get healthy, this time from the starting point of being overweight.

The day seemed to go well early on. I did, after all, finally get to make and enjoy my signature spinach shake once again. This little concoction was my idea of heaven in a cup, designed to start the day off right and keep the hunger pangs away.

Ironically, I also was tasked with coaching in the championship game of the community Little League football team I helped with. What a perfect way to get back into the life of fitness—watching Mini-Me's battling it out on the frozen tundra.

Yet the day slowly became a never-ending parade of reminders of what had been easier times—when I was gaining weight on purpose.

It started when I was running on the field with my team. I didn't make it to the middle of the football field before I was winded. Clearly, just because I decided to be fit didn't mean that my heart, lungs, and body were immediately up to the challenge.

At halftime, one of the kids' moms offered me a steaming cup of hot chocolate. Out of reflex I reached for the cup and was moments away from drinking the delicious treat in one gulp.

The same mom asked, "Isn't this the first day of your Fat2Fit stage?"

I slowly lowered the cup of hot chocolate from my lips, embarrassed and annoyed. First, how could I have nearly slipped just hours in? Second, was she toying with me? Offering a cup of pure chocolate just to see if I'd fold under the pressure?

Next were the hunger pangs that I'd been sure my spinach shake would keep at bay. I wasn't even into the fourth quarter of the game when I could hear and feel my growling stomach. Worse yet, I knew that the snacks awaiting me had nothing to do with a cartoon character baking miniature pieces of cinnamon cereal, and had everything to do with furry greens and crunchy nuts.

The hunger was manageable, in part because I was somewhat prepared; I'd anticipated that problem as I got ready for my big day. But the headaches were a different story. Shortly after we lost the game (perhaps I would have been better as a self-indulging overweight coach?), the pounding began.

With each twinge of pain, the vision of my daily Mountain Dew floated before my eyes. It was calling to me—and probably mocking me—telling me that my body needed the caffeine, required the carbonation. I had never lived through drug-induced withdrawal, but this was the effect of a caffeine headache, and it wasn't pretty.

I persevered. Sticking to my meal plan that first day, I pushed myself through the continued headaches and hunger pains. I tried to convince myself that the healthy food I was eating was more enjoyable than, say, a can of Pringles, and that the absence of sweets and desserts was probably better for my wife and children, too.

When I'd climb the stairs and feel my lungs ache for oxygen, I'd tell myself that tomorrow I'd be a little lighter and the trek wouldn't hurt quite as much. And more than anything else, when I got on the computer and read the stories of the countless individuals in the community who had joined me in pursuing their own health, I felt a sense of both responsibility and accountability.

I remember anticipating that the hardest part of the Fat2Fit stage would be the exercising. I'd feel sore, struggling to do exercises that I had long since perfected, and would probably feel self-conscious at the gym.

After only one day, I realized that the upcoming exercises were the least of my problems. I had to deal with my nutrition, and it wasn't going to be as simple as switching back to "what I'd always eaten." I'd willingly forced my body to accept the diet of a typical, overweight American. Now, as a result, the struggle between what I should eat and what I wanted to eat was going to dominate every single meal.

I'd broken up with Cinnamon Toast Crunch and Mountain Dew. How long did I have to wait until I stopped missing them?

Instant or Long-Term Gratification?

Turn on the television, browse through a magazine, look to the shelves of your local pharmacy, and you're inundated with quick fixes to any potential weight problem. It doesn't matter what the approach is, or who the experts sponsoring it are, the claims are the same: stick to this approach for a short time, and you will see results.

Some diets aim to strike all carbohydrates from your diet, filling you up on only protein. Others provide simple instructions to drink some of your calories, and you'll stop feeling hungry through the majority of the day. Other people swear by eating cabbage soup (or some other specific food) as a way to shed the pounds.

Regardless of the fad, all such approaches share the same inherent flaw—the fact that they're diets. The idea of a diet is straightforward: eat specific "good" foods and restrict yourself from "bad" foods. The problem is that someday (whether it's in a week, a month, or a few hours) "bad" foods will fall back onto your plate. Any progress made will be quickly reversed.

Think back to every diet you've tried. Early on, the going is smooth. The weight starts to drop off as you remove forbidden foods from your diet. Then you start to plateau. Or you're constantly faced with those same foods that your body once used to rely on and are tortured by the temptation.

Gradually, you sneak in one of the forbidden foods, claiming that you'll start dieting again next Monday. Then Monday becomes the *next* Monday, and one forbidden food becomes two—and the initially promising attempt becomes deflating failure.

And yet, whatever the reason for stopping, months after one fad diet has failed you're on the hunt for the next. Before you know it, you're filling your grocery cart with indulgent amounts of cabbage (or whatever), hoping that the answer lies in a never-ending portion of soup or Tabasco sauce or grapefruit juice concoction.

That's the diet side of the health industry. The other side of the equation is the fitness industry. For every quick-fix diet, there's an equally compelling exercise program promising that a few minutes, hours, or routines later you can have the body that you've always dreamed of.

Exercise fanatics believe that hard work at the gym is the real means to long-term weight success. Less dependent on what you're eating, the true change in health, in their view, comes from how many calories are being worked out of your system.

These claims are just as straightforward as those of the diet gurus: put a small amount of work in, and see the results. Only in America could the idea of little effort equating to ridiculous results be embraced as if it were going out of style. How else could you justify the existence of contraptions like the "weight vest" or any variety of metal bars that promise six-pack abs just in time for summer?

The typical exercise-to-lose-weight program takes a similar course to that of fad diets. The initial interest carries results, but a plateau eventually occurs. Or because you're now burning more calories, you also eat more food—and the net result is zero.

For every one of us who's tried a fad diet, we've also tried the quick-fix exercise route. The end result is the reason the health industry is one of the fastest-growing in our nation. Quick-fix exercises don't work, forcing you to go out and try another.

Upon plateau, the exerciser or dieter starts to doubt that those washboard abs or slim thighs are going to come before the next millennium, let alone summer. Dwindling motivation, fading dedication, and busy, busy life start to intervene, and the best-laid plans become just that. Action takes a backseat until next January.

I've always believed that exercise and nutrition go hand in hand. While exercise is important, the key to losing weight and keeping it off lies in what you eat. I'm not talking about a fad diet, though. I'm talking about a nutritional lifestyle change—a holistic approach that takes into account that you will fall off the wagon, eat out at restaurants, and plateau in your journey to lose weight and get healthy. What you eat is the single most important factor in losing weight.

As I stood at the mirror, examining my 70-plus pounds of baggage, I realized that it was critical to share with those who were following me that exercise doesn't get you all the way. It helps, absolutely, but it isn't the critical piece.

> **While exercise is important, the key to losing weight and keeping it off lies in what you eat. I'm talking about a nutritional lifestyle change—a holistic approach that takes into account that you will fall off the wagon, eat out at restaurants, and plateau in your desire to lose weight and get healthy. What you eat is the single most important factor in losing weight.**

So I decided to forgo one of the most important parts of my personal training regimen—working out; I would do only stretching and basic core exercises. I would change my nutrition first, hoping that my results would show that what you put into your system is much more important than anything else when you're trying to lose weight and become healthy.

Unlike the fad diets and workouts that many of us have experienced to some degree (my condolences to all of you), my approach to health is simple. It's my belief that we're all in charge of our own success in finding the path to our health. This approach is a lifestyle, not a diet!

Most approaches require an individual to become almost robotic—eat this, avoid that. What this type of approach fails to consider is that we're human. We're going to struggle, and we're going to make mistakes. And if an approach doesn't make concessions for mistakes and lapses, it's easy to predict the end result: failure.

Many people start exercise and diet routines with the best of intentions, and when they encounter adversity, they quit. Quite simply, quitting is easier than putting in the work. And yet part of the urge to quit is the frustration of feeling like they aren't doing things right or the program isn't working the way they'd hoped.

Besides, when someone else is telling them what to do, it's difficult to own their own decision-making process.

I had always believed that there was an intrinsic choice within everyone—people either chose to be healthy, or they chose not to, and in this way the results spoke for themselves. Becoming overweight provided me with a new reality, a more complicated understanding. I was right that the ability to become healthy was about choice. I was wrong, though, about what the word "choice" meant. I thought that once your mind kicked into gear, everything else would fall into line.

I realized now that nothing was going to simply fall in line for my weight loss. But that's not how I became overweight, either. I had to force myself to start choosing unhealthy foods and behaviors. I had to force myself to eat that first doughnut.

As I started putting on extra pounds, I was making choices multiple times a day—the wrong choices for my health and fitness. Sometime along the journey, however, I stopped having to force myself to choose what was unhealthy. The choices became easy; I'd grown so accustomed to them that I forgot I was making choices—unhealthy ones—every single day. Instead, it just felt like my new routine.

At the end of my six months of weight gain, the concept of choice returned. As I started my way back and began to "eat healthy," I was faced with the same opportunities to make a good or bad choice, not just daily but many times a day. And it was difficult to always choose the right option.

The initial difficulty lay in the headaches from caffeine withdrawal and the urgings of my newfound appetite. Perhaps my body now needed the sugar. Maybe it was the convenience of the processed food. Actually, it was all of the above, and I had to force myself to make the right choice multiple times a day, trusting that the decision making would become easier with time.

I gained 75 pounds in a six-month period by making the wrong choices every day, every hour. I knew that turning away from my new addictions wouldn't be enough. The temptation to make the wrong choice for my health had become a part of me. That temptation would always be just around the corner—every corner. Being healthy is a choice. Getting healthy is an entirely different enterprise that requires a mind shift, a strategy, and a lot of support.

I changed my approach to my daily routine so that when confronted with the opportunity to make choices, I made the right ones. It was the only way to ensure that I continued to move forward in my journey.

Being healthy is a choice. Getting healthy is an entirely different enterprise that requires a mind shift, a strategy, and a lot of support.

Detailed in the pages below are some of the key approaches I used to get back on the path to fitness. These approaches aren't a fad diet; I won't tell you to avoid specific foods at all costs. Getting healthy is about understanding how to make good choices in the face of seemingly more appetizing (but really more damaging) options.

The reality is that we're going to make some wrong choices. But if every day we make a great deal more right choices than wrong, our health will start to change for the better. And then, if we're patient, making the right choices will become automatic—and part of a new routine.

Eat, Drink, Love

When we were growing up, our parents typically used every means necessary to instill life lessons into us. These lessons generally arrived in the shape of books, movies, personal experiences (which tended to involve walking to and from school, uphill, in three feet of snow), and stories.

As children (and especially as teenagers), we would scoff at these apparently trivial stories. We'd perfect the art of rolling our eyes, and our parents would desperately try to find a better analogy to make their point after all.

Little did I know that one of those stories would actually be critical to understanding why we struggle to get out of our unhealthy rut.

Why can't we step away from fast food? Why do we crave processed items at every single meal? The key to answering that question is living through a little story time. (I'll ignore that eye roll!)

One day, a little girl walked into the kitchen to see a large ham sitting on the counter. She crawled onto a stool and watched her mother pull out a knife (don't worry, kids; this isn't a Stephen King novel) and cut the ends off the ham, set the big piece of meat in a pan, and place it in the oven.

The girl was quiet for a long time, a quizzical look on her face. When her mother inquired as to her facial expression, the girl asked about the routine with the ham. "Why did you cut the ends off, Mommy?" she asked.

After a slight pause, her mother stated that it was how her mother had cooked ham. When she was little, it was almost a rite of passage to go through the same steps for the Sunday ham that the family would enjoy. The little girl pressed further: "And why did Grandma cut the ends off?"

Not knowing the answer, the mother picked up the phone and called "Grandma" to inquire. Not surprisingly, the response was very similar—Grandma had witnessed her own mother's approach, and had copied it when she started a family.

Now daughter, mother, and grandmother were curious as to the genesis of their routine. They approached a very elderly great-grandmother and asked, "Why did you cut the ends off a ham before baking it?"

The elderly woman's response was clear and succinct: "Because I had a small pan, and if I hadn't cut it, the ham wouldn't have fit."

Three generations, three inherited routines, and no semblance of logic except in the initial instance. The idea that we do something because that's the way it's always been done seems trite and too convenient until we look at our own lives, especially our own nutrition, and realize that we've fallen into the same patterns.

Ask almost anyone how many meals they should have each day, and the answer will be "three" about 90 percent of the time. Ask them what a proper meal should include, and you'll hear something along the lines of "a meat, a bread, and a side dish."

The Best Spinach Shake Ever

Makes 1 serving

1 scoop Protein2Fit Vanilla Whey Protein Isolate
3 cups fresh spinach
½ banana
2 tablespoons peanut butter (preferably natural)
¾ cup unsweetened almond milk
2 cups ice

Combine these items in a blender, and you're ready to go! This delicious, quick, healthy drink (featured on *The Dr. Oz Show*) is packed with quality protein, good fat, plenty of potassium, a dose of vitamin C, and beneficial fiber. This shake can be used as a great breakfast, lunch, dinner, or pre/postworkout meal; alternatively, you can halve the recipe and enjoy the shake as one of your snacks during the day. To make this extra-low in carbs, omit the banana.

Little do we know that these inherited approaches to nutrition are working against us every single day. The understanding of what "eating healthy" means may have changed over the generations, but our eating habits have not. I'm not going to suggest that the key to proper nutrition is to kick carbs out of your kitchen, or to overdose on protein. The needed changes to nutrition are much subtler than that.

Our bodies need various types of nutrition in order to function well—water, protein, carbohydrates, and fat (yes, fat). All these work together to provide the necessary energy for us to function on a daily basis, and they work with our body's metabolism to burn the proper amount of calories.

I focus on the following areas: I drink plenty of water (enough to have one clear urination per day) and try to stick with foods that are high in fiber, high in protein, low in carbohydrates, and minimally processed. In order to kickstart and maintain a higher metabolism, I also eat every three hours.

Your body needs constant fuel in order to constantly improve and avoid overeating.

People tend to think that protein can be found only in hamburgers and steaks, and that carbohydrates must be procured through breads, pastas, and processed foods. The reality is that the keys of nutrition (protein, carbohydrates, fat) can be found in healthier items.

My meal plans focus on eating a variety of lean meats and legumes (mostly nuts) for protein. These types of protein also provide an adequate amount of fat, killing the need to seek out the fat in a package of Zingers.

Vegetables are an excellent source of carbohydrates and can be eaten without the worry of high calories and fats. It's crucial to understand that carbohydrates fall into two categories—good and bad. The good (high-fiber items) benefit our nutrition. The bad (sugars, refined and processed carbohydrates, etc.) inhibit our progress, and lead to high blood sugar levels, which are linked to a variety of health issues.

And not all liquids are created equal. While we've all been told that eight glasses of water a day is a beneficial, sufficient amount, we tend to seek out interesting ways to get our liquids. Energy drinks, sodas, and fruit juices dominate the market, encouraging us to drink our calories and thus struggle to lose weight. Personally, I found it more enjoyable to drink a liter of Mountain Dew than to down the same amount of water, but by choosing to keep daily calories in the solid foods consumed, as opposed to the Mocha Frappuccinos, we dramatically increase our ability to burn fat and lose weight.

This approach isn't about forcing you to stop eating a certain type of food. It's about helping you realize that a balanced diet needs the same nutritional building blocks as always—and that you can choose to eat healthier items to get the nutrients you need. This is how the pounds come off.

Adopting the Boy Scout Motto

It wasn't a new experience for me to have to commute to and from work each day. In order to get from my home in Utah to the hospital in Idaho in time for work, I'd roll myself out of bed, wolf down some breakfast, grab some snacks and a lunch, and start driving. During the weight-gain phase of my Fit2Fat2Fit journey, though, my pattern changed, with meal stops often added in.

I was a short 30 minutes into the three-hour commute drive one day when I realized I had two problems—first, my smaller-than-usual breakfast, a quick bowl of cereal, wasn't going to sustain me; and second, I had left all of my snacks on the kitchen counter.

A fast trip over to the local McDonald's was the answer. A few Egg McMuffins and orders of hash browns later, my stomach told me I could probably make it to Idaho without further complaints. When I arrived at work and gathered my things to go inside, I realized that my lunch must be sitting next to my pile of snacks back home. I could only imagine the look on Lynn's face when she saw the huge pile of food, resembling the contents of an overfull grocery cart, when she crept down to the kitchen long after I had departed.

My earlier quick escape for the three-hour commute led to a desperate tweet for advice. It was now lunchtime and I was getting hungry. In an ode to every fast-food joint imaginable, my followers gave me a wide range of suggestions (including how I could pull off a midweek food challenge), and I was off to Wendy's for one of their famed Baconators.

After a full day of work, not helped by the array of sweets in the hospital break room, I was ready for the commute home. By the time I pulled into my driveway, a 7-Eleven and Taco Bell had had a friendly visitor drop by.

As I downed what felt like a full bottle of Tums and prepared to go to sleep, I wondered how many calories my forgetful morning had caused. Not that I had healthy snacks in my bag during that phase of my weight adventure, but the trio (a first for me) of McDonald's, Wendy's, and Taco Bell had to have pushed my daily caloric intake into the stratosphere. Needless to say, I took extra time with the stretch-mark lotion before retiring for the evening.

And therein lies one of the great mistakes people make when trying to find nutritional health. No, it's not that I couldn't step away from the fast-food joints. It's that I put myself in a position of unpreparedness.

Mexican Chicken

Makes 4 servings *Prep: 20 minutes* *Cook: 50–60 minutes*

1 pound boneless, skinless chicken breasts
1 teaspoon prepared taco seasoning
½ cup red enchilada sauce
1 small can chopped black olives
1 small can chopped green chilies
4 ounces cheddar cheese, shredded (optional)
3 green onions, chopped

Sprinkle the chicken on both sides with taco seasoning; grill or sauté. Cut the cooked chicken into cubes and place in a greased 8 × 8-inch baking dish. Add the enchilada sauce and toss the chicken to coat. Sprinkle the cheese (optional) and olives over the chicken and bake at 350°F for 10 to 20 minutes, until hot and bubbly. Scatter the green chilies and green onions over the top.

We all need sustenance. If we go long enough, our stomach growls. Wait a bit more, and it feels like our stomach is being eaten alive by the acids inside. By the time we're *really* hungry, we start staring at pets around the house and considering their caloric value.

So when we get hungry and don't have anything around to eat, we seek it out. We search for jars and bowls of candy. We ask our coworkers if they want to split an extra-large pizza.

This is why we all need the Boy Scout motto: "Be prepared."

Every single day we're surrounded by unhealthy foods presented by fast-food companies trying to grab our attention with large portions, quick service, and cheap prices. Those companies know that the key to their business is the window shopper—the person who didn't plan on eating out, but who sees the sign, hears the advertisement, and drops through the drive-through for a quick bite.

In essence, companies selling unhealthy food are trying to get us to cheat on ourselves when we venture out for our day. They want us to give in to our desires. They rely on it.

Being prepared is essential not just for me, but for all of us who want to establish a balanced relationship with food. That's our only defense in the fast-food war.

People don't fall off the wagon because they need a hamburger. More often than not they buy that burger out of a lack of preparation. The key to change is making the right foods just as convenient as (if not more convenient than) the unhealthy options that are thrown in your direction several times every day.

I know we're all busy, and life keeps us from preparing healthy meals from scratch each and every day. With a job and family of my own, I understand the pressure and stress that a busy schedule can bring.

So I simplify things. Twice a week I marinate my meats, cut my vegetables, and cook my meals. I line up a series of containers and create a variety of meals that will serve me for the next three days. Put simply, I get prepared to skip the drive-through.

By preparing my meals in advance, but doing so only twice a week (instead of seven, which is just impractical), I know what I'll eat and how I'll plan. I can guarantee that each meal will keep me going toward my goals—and more important, I make it easy.

A few weeks into the second phase of my journey, Fat2Fit, I found myself facing another Monday commute to Idaho. I pulled myself out of bed (this time, it was much less of a roll!) and went into the kitchen, where I laughed at my wife's support. Placed strategically throughout the kitchen were Post-it notes reminding me to take my cooler. I packed my prepared meals, along with my handpicked snacks, and headed off for the day.

The results were different. No Egg McMuffins this time. No Baconators. No Taco Bell. Why? Because I didn't need to seek sustenance. I enjoyed my prepared meals—good portions of meats and vegetables. And every time I heard my stomach growl, I'd have an option that would quell the hunger, but not at the expense of my health and my waistline.

People don't fall off the wagon because they need a hamburger, specifically. More often than not they buy that burger out of a lack of preparation. The key to change is making the right foods just as convenient as (if not more convenient than) the unhealthy options that are thrown in your direction several times every day.

Go Scouts!

The Potato Skin Shopper

My parents had it easy. They seemed to effortlessly avoid one of the most contentious disagreements ever to grace the great American family—the war over clearing your dinner plate.

I loved fruits and vegetables even as a kid. I loved practically everything my parents put in front of me. While I'll admit that my openness to nutritious food probably had to do with a premature obsession with health, they didn't have to go through staged negotiations to get me to eat dinner, especially living with ten other hungry kids.

In families where vegetables aren't so popular, parents often try to bargain positively (an extra hour of TV or a playdate per successfully eaten serving) or negatively (an earlier bedtime or dropped movie for each portion left untouched). That's quickly followed by the guilt approach: there are starving children who aren't as fortunate as we are, so eat up or the food is going to be shipped to the needy.

If negotiations fail, parents may try making the food artificially exciting. Clearly, a piece of broccoli in flight like an airplane is more appetizing than one sitting quietly next to the mashed potatoes. And finally, when all hope seems lost, there's the nutritional education approach. We're told that we won't grow tall without the vegetables. We're told about the nutritional worth of the skin of a potato.

I remember eating baked potatoes as I grew up, and I didn't care for the skin. It was chewy, and did I mention that it was brown? My parents tried to convince me that the warm, fluffy interior actually held no nutritional value. It was all in the skin, which would help me to keep up with my taller and more athletic brothers and sisters.

Years later, I performed my own version of MythBusters research to find out whether the claims regarding potato skins were true or false. (If I'm about to shatter one of the great lessons that your parents taught you, I apologize in advance.) The bottom line? A potato's food value lies as much in the delicious white interior as it does in the scruffy brown skin!

Fast-forward to the grocery store, as I got ready to buy the right foods for my journey back to health. A display of potatoes caught my eye, and I realized that my own lesson in health could be shared via my parents' claims regarding the potato skin. Hold that thought for a moment.

It took 75 extra pounds for me to realize that the simple choice of becoming healthy was only the beginning of a very difficult journey.

One of the key necessities in developing a healthy lifestyle is to realize what's bad for you—and generally, if it tastes too good to be true, it probably is. American industry and culture have, over the years, perfected the trade of processed foods that we all crave. Where would we be without our boxed mac and cheese, for example?

Even when we accept the reality that processed foods are working against us and our health, it's difficult to step away. And the problem starts at the grocery store. Walking in after a long day at work, you're faced with 15 to 20 aisles of goodness. These stores have the best deals and cheapest foods right in the middle of the store, so once you've headed down an aisle, it's like you've already lost the battle.

What started as a "Can you pick up milk?" trek to the grocery store turns into a 45-minute stroll up and down every aisle, with a cartful of junk as a reward. As the weeks pass by, even those of us trying to shop wisely wonder why we aren't healthy—and, more importantly, why the fruits and veggies in the fridge have started to rot.

While my parents pulled a fast one on me with the potato skin myth, I'm not one to let something go to waste. In the time-honored tradition of turning "lemons" into lemonade, I actually use this false myth to solve the grocery store dilemma. It can also help you to focus on the right types of foods (lean meats, nuts, seeds, fruits, vegetables). Who said Mom and Dad's little white lies wouldn't come in handy?

I want you to envision your local grocery store as a large potato. The back wall and the aisles on the far sides of the building are the skin. The middle aisles are the white, fluffy goodness that we love. Please note: the skin is where you need to stay. Avoid the middle at all costs.

The outside edges of the store are absolute nirvana to a life of health. Here you'll find fruits, vegetables, lean meats, healthy seafood, and excellent sources of protein. And while it's true that your local grocery store isn't going to have a "10 Fillets of Salmon for $10!" sale anytime soon, you'll save much more important things, namely your resolve, self-esteem, and health.

So for now, I'll forgive my parents for their small fib about potato skins. After all, the more you view your weekly shopping experience as eating that outside part of the potato, the closer you'll be to your goals.

It seems that the world challenges your good nutritional intentions at every turn.

It would be easier if you could text-message the entire world, asking everyone to support your life decisions. How wonderful would it be to walk into a grocery store that carried only healthy foods? I truly believed, back in my fit days, that once the decision to lose weight and become healthy was made, the will to follow meal plans and workout routines would naturally become the new routine.

Spinach Egg-White Omelet

Makes 1 serving

½ cup egg whites (from about 3 large eggs) and 1 whole egg
¼ cup chopped onions
2 tablespoons chopped jalapeños (optional)
½ cup fresh spinach
¼ cup chopped mushrooms
¼ cup chopped red bell pepper
½ cup precooked chicken breast
2 tablespoons salsa

Spray a medium-size skillet with olive oil nonstick spray. Mix the egg whites and whole egg together. Once the pan reaches medium-high heat, add the eggs and wait 30 seconds. Then add the onions, jalapeños, spinach, mushrooms, red bell pepper, and chicken breast, placing them in a line along the middle. Once the eggs start to bubble and become firm on the bottom (usually 1 to 2 minutes), indicating that the omelet is ready to flip, sprinkle the outside edges with water using your fingertips—as it bubbles it creates a space that helps make it easier to use a spatula for flipping. Flip/close the omelet and cook for another minute or so; then flip the omelet to the other side for another 1 to 2 minutes, or until done. Once the omelet is cooked to your liking, serve with the salsa on top and enjoy.

It took 75 extra pounds for me to realize that the simple choice of becoming healthy was only the beginning.

What came next was learning to deal with the constant barrage of choices that had to be made in order to support my approach to nutrition. When I stopped at the gas station for a fill-up, I had to remind myself not to pick up Zingers, but to eat from my bag of healthy treats. And, as I mentioned earlier, twice a week I used my evenings to prepare meals ahead, making the difficult choices a little bit easier.

And things did get easier. The second day, while immensely difficult, was a bit easier to handle than the first. The second week continued to barrage me with choices, but my resolve and willpower seemed to be equal to the task.

As I explained earlier, the personal trainer in me decided not to exercise during the first month of Fat2Fit. While I was hopeful that careful eating would pull me through, little did I know that sheer nutrition could lead to such overwhelming results.

In six months, I had gained 75 pounds. In one month of proper nutrition, I lost 19. My body fat dropped by 5 percent, and my energy level skyrocketed. My testosterone level almost doubled (249 to 475), my total cholesterol went from 147 to 116, my LDL (bad cholesterol) went from 80 to 62, my triglycerides went from 132 to 59, and my insulin level went from 51 to 5 (normal).

Was it as simple as making a single choice and watching the results flow in? Sadly, no. I'd simplified the world so much as a personal trainer that I was blind to the reality of how difficult this process can be.

But there's another reality. Every choice presented to us is an opportunity. And every day, we have 10, 20, 30 opportunities to make the right choice. The key is being prepared, which makes every right choice that much easier. It worked for me. Losing 19 pounds without lifting a weight or doing a push-up was better than I'd expected.

Unfortunately, my journey to becoming fit would involve more than just nutrition, and all that fun stuff was still to come . . .

CHAPTER 6

THE GYM MEMBERSHIP THAT WON'T GO TO WASTE

There was something sinister in his smile. Sure, he had been a supportive friend as I had gained over 70 pounds, but now that I was on my way back, his smile didn't match the current conversation.

I was in the middle of lunch with one of my closest friends, and I had just finished relating my sense of nervousness about the coming week—the first time that I would start working out in seven months. And all he did was slyly smile, as if he was enjoying my unease. His expression conveyed a single thought: payback.

When I was a personal trainer, taking on a new client was always an interesting prospect. Taking on a client who also happened to be a family member or a friend complicated matters, as I noted when talking about James.

After all, one of the key characteristics of a good personal trainer is to push "trainees" to accomplish what they can't on their own. And being strangers helps this—as the trainer, you feel less guilty about really engaging them, and you're far enough removed from their bad habits or poor routines that it doesn't frustrate you.

Family and friends, however, challenge you in a different way. They're usually much more honest about their struggles and breakdowns, but they also have an underlying expectation that the bond you share will guarantee results (no doubt with half the effort!).

Months before the idea of Fit2Fat2Fit had even entered my brain, the friend in question had asked me to take him under my wing and provide some personal training. I agreed, with a mix of excitement and trepidation. His would be an interesting training regimen, as he wasn't overweight but simply wanted to build and tone muscle.

I suggested that we work out at a gym so that I could have the full arsenal of equipment at my disposal. He politely declined, asking to be trained in the comfort of his own basement. That response caught me off guard. I had seen how fear of the gym had held overweight clients back, but this friend had nothing to be embarrassed about.

I found myself feeling slightly bemused at some of his difficulties as I took him through the paces of his first workout. Starting out, the problems were simple enough—he needed some extra water breaks, and he frequently mentioned that he "hadn't worked out like this . . . ever." I was patient, but persistent. I was going to get him to work his body like never before.

Then came complaints about, of all things, his nose going numb! As a personal trainer, I had heard every excuse in the book, but a numbing nose in the middle of a 45-minute workout? I had my doubts. This was followed by pangs of nausea that he said were coming on stronger with every exercise. After another, lengthier break, I encouraged him to keep it up. Halfway through the next set of push-ups, he sprinted to the bathroom and vomited. End of workout.

As a good friend and personal trainer, I called him the next day to see if he would even consider letting me back into his basement to continue to train. While he said he was still game, he also commented that our single workout had caused bizarre behaviors—like walking down the stairs backward. Apparently he was so sore he couldn't walk down the stairs like a normal human being. The pain was too severe.

The soreness was winning the war. And sadly, I thought it was as convincing as the nose that went numb. The excuses and complaints were piling up faster than the push-ups.

We lasted only two more sessions. While no other experience involving vomit took place, the nose of constant numbing made numerous returns, and the slight tension between trainer and trainee continued to build. He graciously ended our agreement.

So as I drove home from that lunch many months (and 75 pounds) later, I smiled at my friend's reaction to my impending workout routines. He was clearly going to enjoy my struggle with the exercise portion of my journey back to fitness. And I was eager to prove that his experience was just another example of someone not doing enough to get the fitness he desired.

Two days later, as I pulled into a parking space in front of the gym, I hesitated. For the first time in my life, I was actually nervous to go in. What would people think when they saw me, overweight and struggling through basic moves? After all, *my* picture was on the wall, advertising my Fit2Fat-2Fit journey.

Getting into the gym, rough though it was, was the easy part. Apparently, doing a single set of push-ups was more than my body could handle. Halfway through my first exercise group, I couldn't get over the sensation of my stomach hitting the mat, and my knees buckled to the floor. I was doing knee push-ups, and just barely surviving.

After every set of reps, my arms were shaking (slightly at first, violently by the end). I kept glancing around, wondering what judging eyes could be watching me. I pressed on, though, and made it through my first workout in seven months.

At least I didn't vomit, I thought as I headed home, physically shaken and mentally defeated. It was a struggle to admit to my wife that knee push-ups had been required and that so much strength had been lost in such a short period of time.

The worst of it came the next day. I knew I was in trouble when the pain in my chest and arms actually woke me up. Getting out of bed, I felt like knives were stabbing into my muscles, and the staircase to the kitchen looked like it was 300 miles long.

The personal trainer in me rationalized it as a condition called DOMS (delayed-onset muscle soreness). However, as I took every step as slowly as humanly possible, and actually cried out in pain when I picked up my two-year-old, my friend's face came into focus.

To me, the pain might have been DOMS. To him, and to many of my previous clients, it was something else: payback.

Secrets of a Good Exercise Routine

It's truly amazing what you can find on television in the dead of night when you can't sleep. No, the airwaves aren't filled with trashy movies, second-rate reality shows, or sports bloopers. Every single minute from about 1:00 A.M. to 5:00 A.M. is filled with something slightly more intoxicating—infomercials.

There are 30-minute specials on every product imaginable. If you struggle with acne, weight, rotting food, a shortage of fresh pasta, stains on your carpet, or even a lack of hair, the late-night infomercials are a one-stop shop. If you call within the next 15 minutes, you get even more amazing deals!

One night, early in my Fat2Fit journey, I couldn't sleep and found myself surfing through these infomercials. I stumbled upon a series of specials about exercise. After about two hours of being sold to, even the personal trainer in me was convinced that I could lose my 70-plus pounds of extra weight by barely lifting a finger.

The first special I watched made things seem terribly easy. All I had to do was put 10 minutes in per day, and the weight would come off. There were no special diets, and I wasn't required to put in hours at the gym. Even better, there was no special equipment. By following an exercise routine that provided roughly an hour of physical activity a week, I'd lose inches and pounds. Really!

That was followed by what can only be described as a human torture device—one that could conveniently be stored under your bed when not in use, and firmly attached to the back of any normal bedroom door when needed. The key, it appeared, was that regular exercise didn't do enough. However, by doing the same routines while bolted into a fancy (and costly) contraption, I'd lose inches and pounds. If that wasn't enough, I was introduced to a much less costly and intimidating contraption—one that ensured

I was doing a proper abdominal crunch every time. Contrary to popular belief, I was told, the only thing holding me back from rock-hard abs (that glisten in the sun) was a five-minute routine. I didn't have to lift weights or do hours of cardio; all I had to do was buy the video and the bar and I'd lose inches and pounds. Yes, really!

As I was getting ready to fall asleep, I was greeted with one final infomercial. Taking a completely different tack, this was hard-core: 12 individual workouts, six days a week. I would be working out one to two hours a day on this regimen, and it would be the hardest thing I'd ever done. This would be like having a personal trainer at my house every single day, I was told. If it didn't physically kill me, I'd be the talk of the town. But just to show that it wasn't too cumbersome, I was promised that it would take only three months to find the best shape of my life. If I bought the entire package, I'd lose pounds and inches pronto.

I couldn't tell if I was exhausted because it was 4:00 A.M. or because these infomercials became harder to believe. Yet I was awake enough to realize that all of the infomercials had three critical parts to their pitch:

Go extreme. None of the specials mentioned the importance of balance and realism. Instead, your choices were to do as little as possible for amazing results (with the product), or sacrifice your lifestyle and body for amazing results (without the product).

Shh! It's a secret! Only after you spent $50 or more could you learn the secret to a better you. Doing only basic exercises or routines wasn't adequate. You would never reach your true potential. You needed a special video, contraption, or human torture device—available only from this one source.

There's no other option. Like any good sales message, the presentations made it clear that the only way to true health and fitness was contained in the infomercial. There was no customization to an individual's interests, abilities, or desires. If you followed the scripted and convoluted plan, you would lose weight, with the consistent reminder that "results may vary."

In truth, exercise and fitness have very little to do with secret components. They're about other important aspects—persistence, balance, and interest.

If changing nutritional habits is all about making the right choices each hour and day, appropriate fitness and exercise are about persistence—pulling yourself off the couch every single day to get physical activity. In some ways, a change in nutrition is easier, because you're presented with so many opportunities to self-correct or get back on the wagon. Exercise is more difficult, and typically more intrusive on our busy lives. Between a job, family, children, friends, and other activities, who has the time, energy, and patience to fit in a two-hour workout? Yet making the time to ensure we get enough physical activity is crucial to finding fitness and health.

Moreover, the necessary and most critical approach to an exercise routine is balance. Sure, results can be found in the most extreme of programs. These will push the body and mind to depths and lengths they never expected to go. And sure, there are select individuals who can get away with just 10 minutes of exercise every day and still maintain a high metabolism and good figure. But true fitness is about balance—putting the time, effort, and energy into a workout, but only to the point of feeling a healthy tension. The body is a machine—it needs to be worked, and it needs downtime. When damaged, it needs breathers to repair and revitalize. Finding the right place between too little and too much is critical to developing a sound exercise philosophy and approach.

Finally, an appropriate exercise mind-set focuses on individual interests. We can't be good at, or enjoy, every activity put in front of us. For the same reason that some of us love seafood and others run for the hills when it's put in front of us, the specific form of exercise must hold a person's interest. Because believe me, there will come a time when you won't want to put in the time and effort required. If you have no interest in the type of exercise routine you're doing, you'll stop at that point. And so will your path to health.

When people looked at pictures of me taken before the journey began, they would often ask how I was able to fit in what must have taken two or three hours of exercise a night. They assumed that it was impossible to get my results by powering through a 45-minute workout four or five times a week at the local gym or in the basement.

I'm not sure they believed me when I told them the truth. Like them, I said, I had work, a family, and friends. What I didn't have was an extra three hours of free time. I had achieved fitness through workouts of 45 minutes to an hour, four or five times a week. And I did so with the proper mix of persistence, balance, and interest.

As I slogged my way back into the gym after seven months of inactivity, however, I finally realized just how foreboding and scary the mountain looked when you were at the bottom. Getting out of the routine of lazy nights on the couch was brutal, and I often considered taking a night or two off, just because I felt ineffective. I mean, I couldn't do a regular push-up anymore. What would it matter if I relaxed for just one evening?

The answer was simple: because health and fitness aren't found on the couch. They're found at the gym, in a workout room, or outside, and they're found with the right mind-set. And so I pushed myself back to the gym, day after day, remembering that the key was balance; I didn't need to kill myself.

I knew that to get in great shape and maintain my fitness would take persistence, balance, and exercise that held my interest. And, as with my approach to nutrition, I needed a plan that I could follow. Yet a plan wasn't going to be enough. There were pitfalls ahead—dangers that could derail even the most ardent, focused individual—and it was important to know what was coming and how to stay on track and keep moving forward.

Everything I Know About Balance

There are many rites of passage as a person grows out of childhood and into adulthood. For the socially conscious, the first time you enter a voting booth is the true indication that you're now someone to be taken seriously.

For others, it's a quick trip to a casino to gamble or pull the handle of a slot machine that signifies youth is gone and an open world of opportunity lies before you.

My rite of passage was getting my driver's license. At that moment the virtual umbilical cord was severed from my parents, and I was suddenly able to go to the mall, the grocery store, or a movie without having to beg my mom to drop me off (albeit half a block from the entrance, so I wouldn't be seen by my friends).

I can't have been the only person who took driver's education more seriously than all my other schooling. I was determined to pass my driving test on the first try and wanted to run down to the DMV as soon as my . . . mom could take me.

Leading up to driver's education, I remember watching my parents drive. It seemed so simple. You twisted the steering wheel a little, turned on the blinker now and then, and hit the gas when the light turned green. I was unable and unprepared to drive at that point, and had no idea what it took to safely navigate the neighborhood, but that didn't stop me from thinking I knew better.

Driver's education changed that. Through supervised road tests (with other fearful students), the reality of just what it took to drive a car came into view. I seemed to have a bad habit of scaring my fellow passengers and my instructor whenever I took to the road. And as I learned how to operate one foot between the gas pedal and the brake (the two-footed driving I'd been imagining apparently wasn't acceptable), check my blind spots, and parallel park, I realized just how incompetent I was at driving a car. No matter how many times I read the driving manual, I clearly wasn't grasping how to make the car go without risking the lives of those around me.

Then came the big day of the test—which I passed!—and subsequent trips out and about on my own. It was white-knuckle driving at its best. My body was tense the whole time. I checked my blind spots so much that I developed new blind spots right in front of the car; and it felt best to go 10 miles under the speed limit just to be safe. Just a day or two after I got my license, I took a quick trip over to the local grocery store, which was only 10 minutes away. By the time I arrived, I was exhausted. I was doing absolutely everything I should while operating the car, and the process took my full concentration and effort.

I'm not sure how long the adjustment took, but my level of comfort with an automobile is slightly different these days. Like most Americans, I've found that I can drive the car, eat a sandwich, tune the radio, and sometimes even check my text messages, leaving only the occasional moment to check my blind spots. Please know that I'm working to change these bad habits. And yet I drive so "unconsciously" these days that I sometimes reach my destination without remembering how I got there (or worrying about who I might have run off the road)!

In other words, as my experience grew in operating an automobile, my comfort level grew as well. Soon I was doing things with a car that I'd never dreamed of on my first day of driver's education class. In truth, I can't say whether I'm a good or a bad driver—I don't really think about it. But I've certainly picked up some lazy and bad habits along the way.

As I drive down the road writing this book (just kidding, Mr. Officer), it's painfully clear to me that a lot of us approach exercise the same way that we learn to drive a car—and the end result is a lack of overall accomplishment (along with some of those pesky bad habits).

Prior to exercise, it's easy to look at people in control of their fitness, and say, "Why can't I do that?" It seems so basic to be able to do a push-up or a pull-up, and running on a treadmill is just running in place, isn't it? Everyone else can do it, so why not me? Why not now? In truth, the blood, sweat, and tears required to start shaping one's body into a fine, well-oiled machine is difficult to understand until it's experienced firsthand.

Each year those of us with any connection to the fitness world see the same ritual. After a guilt-ridden holiday season, droves of people purchase a gym membership and make a resolution to head faithfully to the gym. For some months they make a valiant effort.

These "resolutioners" are easy to spot. They're the ones who can't figure out how to turn on the latest treadmill-like machine; they stand in front of it looking at it as if it were a relic from the Inquisition, used for torture as opposed to exercise. Their effort needs to be applauded; they're on the right track. But as these folks work their way through exercise routines, not sure

The Essential Exercises: Hand Step-Ups with Plank

STEP 1 **Place a low step against a wall for stability, or use your stairs at home.**

STEP 2 **Now get in push-up position on the floor, facing the step in front of you.**

STEP 3 **Put one hand flat on the top of the step, followed by the other hand (keeping your body in a straight line—hence the word "plank").**

STEP 4 **Return hands down off the step/stair one at a time until you're back in the starting push-up position.**

Repeat these movements, at a fast pace, for approximately 30 to 45 seconds, depending on your fitness level. If you're a beginner, you can do this exercise on your knees until you build up the strength to do it without the added assistance. This is a great exercise that works your core, shoulders, and arms and also gets your heart rate up; this combination helps you to burn fat and build muscle at the same time.

if they're accomplishing anything, their first bursts of motivation begin to wane.

Many resolutioners make it through this tough first stage with sheer determination and move on to what I call the competent stage, where individuals have learned to use the various pieces of equipment properly. Their bodies are most likely not ready for the onslaught of punishment, however. They hit 20 push-ups, and it feels as if their chest is going to explode. After an hour passes, they can barely pull themselves home, wondering if their body can take the next visit. Even days later they can still feel every single rep of every single move. The pain of the competent stage is a barrier that forces some resolutioners away for good and, for others, saps even more of their initial drive and motivation.

Yet the strong and determined march on. Results are beginning to show, and the effort seems to be paying off.

A couple of months pass, and those same 20 push-ups are now easy. The treadmill is so comfortable that its inhabitant is focused more on finding the right television show to watch than on anything to do with his or her body.

Then something strange happens: the results stop. Tireless exercisers who reach this level are now frustrated, and the effort spent at the gym doesn't seem to be worthwhile. The workouts fly by so easily that these people don't really remember what exercises they did. Without results, though, a new boredom and a sense of failure creep in. Without physical improvement and soreness to prove they're working hard, exercisers stop making visits to the gym. Now when they think about the gym, the frustration is more about their gym membership fee being wasted.

In this annual ritual, we can see the inherent problem with so many of our efforts to get healthy. Like teenagers learning to drive a car, our bodies figure things out. Before you know it, your body has adjusted to the pain, soreness, and fatigue of exercise because it's getting stronger. In just a few short weeks, you're flying through routines that you didn't think you could possibly survive. The result is called a plateau. Your body gets used to the same movements, weights, and cardio routines; it learns to unconsciously survive the daily trip to the gym, without any threat of DOMS lurking around the corner.

The key to fitness is to confuse your body so that it continues to progress. In other words, you need to be smarter than your body, and always one step ahead. It's imperative to switch up your workout routine every two to four weeks. Choosing different cardio equipment, weight, intensity of exercise, or fitness classes forces your body to readjust. And in that readjustment, the ongoing results are found. The more that you can keep your body from feeling comfortable, the more energy you will expend, resulting in greater weight loss and muscle mass.

If you find yourself not feeling sore, it's because your body is adjusting. It's getting used to the routine and doesn't need to burn as many calories. If doing 20 push-ups is now child's play, push it to 40, add a pulse, or perform them on a medicine ball. If 30 minutes of power walking on the treadmill barely gets you winded, kick it up to a slow run.

Your body will never get comfortable if you follow this strategy, and the results will be startling. And because the results will pile up, the will to continue to fight for those results won't be lost.

If you treat every single exercise routine as if you were a clueless teenager trying to figure out how to operate a car, you'll be surprised at just how far you can push your body—certainly much farther than the 20 push-ups that nearly killed you just days or weeks before.

This change-up approach has a dual effect. Not only does it prevent us from reaching a plateau and losing interest, it also eliminates the boredom from the workout. Our initial motivation gets bolstered as we feel ourselves getting stronger. We begin to witness tangible results in the way we look and feel. Soon the gym is no longer an enemy to be avoided. We've created a gym experience that's sustainable, an approach to fitness that won't fade by March.

Finding Your Own Balance

Even though I am one, I can fully admit that men are interesting creatures when it comes to relationships. Very early on, a lot of men realize that any good relationship is about control, and we go through various stages of trying to wrestle away a little more.

First comes the predating power grab. We men spend countless hours perfecting the most blush-inducing pickup lines, and after a single date begin to play the game. There are rules to be followed—how quickly to call after a date, how much to spend on dinner (or, if you're unsure, just stick to a quick coffee or soda). We think we're in control, that we're dictating next steps.

But then we wake up to find ourselves in a three-month relationship, realizing that we're supposed to (and do) call her every night before bed. We make sure she gets where she needs to go, and in the effort of trying to maintain a level of decision-making ability, start to give in to activities like "chick flicks."

By the time the relationship is serious, we've fully given up even the pretense that we're in control of where the relationship is going. Our only true ability to control something is to find subtle ways to avoid the "define the relationship" or "what kind of ring?" talks.

Even everyday activities like shopping for new clothes take on a whole new meaning. Instead of thinking that the brown pants–black shirt ensemble is just a cute personality quirk, she's redesigning our wardrobe, making sure that we're at least "presentable" to family and friends.

Before we know it, marriage arrives, and although we won't openly admit it, all control has been ceded to the wife. The house is decorated in her style, the social calendar is filled with "double dates," and we spend a little too much time arguing about the best baby name in the world.

So in my version of this scenario, I did what any self-respecting married man would do—I clung to as many activities as I could from my single days. I watched insane amounts of football, went on long hikes, and went mountain biking, and strategically scheduled get-togethers with my male friends to do "manly" things like . . . watch football or go hiking. It was the only thing I had left to show that I was still myself. It was my little bit of comfort.

Yet the gentle prodding and "sculpting" from my wife continued. She constantly made sure I was dressing appropriately (enough). She pulled me out to fine restaurants to help me understand that chicken fajitas weren't the only food in this world. We experienced the theater, movies that actually made me cry (but I'll deny it regardless), and participated in cultural events that opened my eyes to new and fascinating parts of the world.

Somewhere along the line, it hit me: Lynn had actually improved me. As much as I had tried to wrestle control away, and to dictate where things were headed, I now marveled at the person I had become. I dressed much better than anyone who knew me years ago would have expected. I was cultured, well rounded, and the experiences and lessons I'd learned had helped to make a better me.

This is something I never could have done on my own—I needed to be forced to try things that I'd never even considered. And the results have been more positive and more impactful than I would have imagined in my single days.

If only our spouses could influence our approach to health and fitness in the same way! When left to our own devices, we're lost souls, and decidedly less well rounded than we need to be.

Look at individuals around you, and look at yourself. Ask anyone what their favorite type of exercise is, and they'll give you a clear answer. You have your runners, who seem to shy away from any sort of weight machine and would rather spend hours traveling tens of miles in the open air (even in the rain) than put in a good workout at the gym.

Swimmers tend to be similarly focused. They hate running with a passion and would rather live in water to get their proper exercise, spurning every gym option but the pool.

The weight-lifting crew are masters of their local gym. Everyone knows everyone else, and it's a constant competition to see who can lift more, do more, and sweat more. Yet those folks look at the treadmills on the "cardio" side of the gym with bewilderment—how could anyone actually want to run in place for 45 minutes when you could be pumping iron?

Those who seriously participate in yoga look down on the exercising "commoners" and our clearly broken chi. They can do things with their bodies that most people would expect to see only at the local circus, yet the idea of performing "lawnmowers" or "butterflies" with 50-pound weights would do something sinister to their own energy.

And let's not forget the fitness-class alumni. Whether it be light weight lifting, extreme cardio, abdominal workouts that last for a day and a half, or even dance moves that embarrass any male participant, the routines of these alumni are established, and they wouldn't even consider doing something as uninteresting as swimming laps or running down a street.

That's not to say that being an expert in one of these types of exercise isn't fantastic. Any sort of consistent exercise routine will help any individual take steps toward health and fitness.

The Essential Exercises: Dumbbell Squats with a Pulse, Followed by Dumbbell Military Press

STEP 1 With dumbbells held resting on your shoulders, get in position with your knees shoulder-width apart.

STEP 2 Go down until your butt is parallel to the floor; then come up about a quarter of the way.

STEP 3 Go all the way back down to your parallel position and come all the way up.

STEP 4 On the way up, lift the dumbbells above your head until your arms are extended all the way.

STEP 5 Bring dumbbells back to the starting position (resting on your shoulders) before you start your next rep.

But gaining well-rounded fitness and health requires a more balanced approach. Prior to starting my journey, many friends believed that I was a "meathead": they thought I lived at the gym, religiously using every weight available, and showing off just how much weight I could bench. But weight training was only part of my approach to fitness. Accepting that a balanced mix of different exercise routines was going to help me achieve my goals—an acceptance I reached before I became a trainer—was much easier to embrace and support than was giving up my wardrobe choices to my wife.

In addition to weight training, I engaged in running, cardio, swimming, exercise classes, and yes, even yoga. When friends would find out that I was making sure I had time for my "downward dog," they would scoff, thinking that something was clearly off balance. But the reality is that our bodies need different types of workout. Just as we discussed in the section on how to avoid the plateau, following a well-rounded workout routine challenges your body in different ways, providing an even and distinct set of results.

Weight training is vital to help you work muscles in a controlled setting and focus on tightening up what can easily become loose over time. Running, cardio, and swimming are excellent ways to burn a higher number of calories, stripping away persistent fat and driving down overall BMI (body mass index—calculated from a person's height and weight). Yoga focuses heavily on breathing, stretching, and flexibility—three critical pieces to being able to reach a higher level of accomplishment.

All of these different physical gains are beneficial, and you can't get them all from a single type of workout. Perhaps most important, a balanced and well-rounded approach to fitness, incorporating *all* of these approaches, keeps things interesting and thus keeps you working out.

It takes a very patient and persistent person to get on a treadmill and run multiple miles, every single day. The same goes for the person who lifts weights every day for an hour, or swims the equivalent of five miles in the pool. Unless you are lucky (or, as my wife would attest, unlucky) enough to have the obsessive health-nut gene, there will come a time that your typical exercise routine grows stale. That's the time to mix things up and challenge your body with new exercise approaches that you may never have considered.

When I look back at how I was prior to dating, courting, and marrying my wife, I realize how much tunnel vision I truly had regarding life as a whole. I had my routines, approaches, and likes, and I was happy to stick with them. Without a kick in the rear from Lynn, I wouldn't have looked around me to see all the fantastic things there are to do and discover. I credit my wife for any self-actualization that I've accomplished, because she continued to push me into experiences I never would have tried on my own.

To reach true fitness and health, we need to become self-actualized health nuts, willing to dip our toes into a variety of exercise types. The well-rounded and balanced exerciser will not only find greater results, but will be able to continue to have exercise be a part of daily life without things ever getting so stale that the only alternative is to stop exercising altogether.

Form Matters

Sports. For males, it's the great bridge, the one subject that never fails when conversation wanes. Sports also provides the only real occasions where men can jump up and down and act like maniacs and get away with it. Sports can easily become an obsession that determines our moods. If you don't believe me, hang out with a guy who just witnessed his favorite team losing their biggest game—yeah, it's not pretty.

So whenever Tom and I were knee-deep in conversation about sports, everything seemed right in the world. That is, until he brought up the four-letter word that instills fear, anger, and despair in even the most accomplished or gifted athlete—golf.

I'm terrible at golf. It's easier to admit it right out of the gate than to try to rationalize that everyone is bad at the sport. No, golf isn't my strong suit. Give me a football and I'm like a fish in water. Give me a club and a golf ball, and I hit the proverbial wall—hard.

Tom, apparently, was equally woeful. But he was more persistent than I ever was with the sport. After a few failed rounds of golf, I'd given it up as a bad job. He kept coming back to golf, no matter how ugly things got.

To try to learn how to play well, my friend decided to take official lessons. Clearly, spending hours at a driving range, hitting a fair share of "worm burners," wasn't reaping rewards, so it was time to bring in a professional. I admit that my curiosity was piqued. Although I wasn't planning on picking the sport up again anytime soon, I was interested to hear any secrets or tips that were shared.

The lesson, however, was unexpected. The instructor sat back and watched Tom hit a bucket of 50 balls. At any given moment, my friend was expecting that the tips and tricks would start flowing. Yet not a word was shared. Finally, after a full bucket of balls, Tom turned to the instructor and asked, "So what's my problem?" Forgetting to "be careful what you wish for," my friend was inundated with "tips."

Apparently, Tom never approached the ball the same way. He was inconsistent in his practice swings. Furthermore, his practice swings didn't match his real ones. His grip was wrong, sometimes too soft and other times too strong. He didn't pivot his hips, he pivoted them too much, he looked up instead of watching the ball, and he had improper follow-through.

When Tom asked if there was anything slightly salvageable, the instructor smiled and said he had a nice set of golf clubs. When pushed as to how he could start turning around his golf game, the instructor was more forthcoming.

In general, the problem was the form of the swing. He had the right equipment, and the actual swing wasn't terrible. But until he started perfecting the form, and focusing more on hitting the ball right (as opposed to becoming a professional golfer on the PGA circuit), the results would be less than ideal and his frustration would only increase.

Despite my own failed attempts at golf and my decision that nothing good could come from the sport, golf did give me a new perspective. As I continued my journey back from Fat2Fit, I realized that every time I entered the gym I was surrounded by individuals who were taking the same approach to fitness that my friend had to golf.

We see the "golfing" exercisers every day. Many times, we are the "golfing" exercisers. There's the person on the treadmill, clearly running too fast for her current level. To compensate, she's gripping the sides of the machine or dangerously placing her feet on the sides of the treadmill to catch her breath.

Not far away, you'll find the biceps curler. Clearly overdoing it, instead of a smooth and natural lifting of dumbbells, he uses centrifugal force and every back muscle possible to swing the weights to his chest. It would be much better to use less weight and get the form right than to buckle his knees and back in an attempt to lift the weight.

And a little way down from him is the expert cruncher. If you listen quietly, you can hear the counting nearing a hundred, yet on closer examination the head is the only part of the exerciser's body actually moving. You're not sure what muscles are being worked, but you're quite sure that the abdominal region isn't being affected at all. (Perhaps this person is working to build stronger neck muscles?)

The Essential Exercises: Dumbbell Push-Ups with Dumbbell Rows

STEP 1 Start in push-up position, with your hands not flat on the floor but grasping dumbbells placed on the ground about shoulder width apart. (You can do this on your knees if needed.)

STEP 2 With legs spread wide apart go down, do a push-up, and come back to the top.

STEP 3 At the top, pull up one of the dumbbells and do a dumbbell row, keeping the dumbbell and your arm close to your body.*

STEP 4 After the dumbbell row, lower your weight slowly back to the ground, resuming the starting position.

STEP 5 Follow that with another push-up; and this time, at the top of the push-up, do a dumbbell row with the other hand.

Alternate arms after each push-up set.

---

* Pull one dumbbell up to your side until it makes contact with ribs or until your upper arm is just beyond horizontal.

Three examples that can be witnessed in every gym in America, every single day—and one reality. It's not enough just to exercise. It's not good enough to do hundreds of reps. You need to do them right. You need proper form. Otherwise, you're just like the bad golfer—swinging incessantly and not getting better in the slightest.

A lack of proper form has a variety of causes. For some, it's a lack of knowledge. They were never taught proper technique, so they do the best that they can. For others, there's a desire to do more than they can handle, caused by either peer or internal pressure to perform. Still, for others it's the belief that more good will come from three hours in the gym than from one, no matter what the technique.

The truth, however, is quite different. It's not enough that you've made the decision to exercise and do it consistently. It's of great importance to learn how to do each exercise, and to focus on proper mechanics and movements rather than trying to set a weight-lifting or cardio record.

If people exercise with improper form, the desired results will not come. Worse still, potential injury is a real possibility. And more importantly, both injury and lack of results lead to individuals dropping exercise routines and getting farther away from the health and fitness they desire.

Equally important is understanding what typical exercise lingo actually means. An individual can be doing too much or too little because they don't know the difference between a "set" and a "rep." The number of times that you perform an exercise represents the number of sets. The number of times that you lift each weight represents the number of reps, or repetitions. The combination of proper form and knowledge helps even the most inexperienced gym "rookie" to reach new heights.

When you engage in a new routine, it's important that you do your homework and analyze the movements, routines, and exercises that you will participate in. It's better to do a single set of reps properly than it is to do double sets the wrong way. And as your body grows stronger, it will tell you clearly when it's time to increase the intensity and resistance. For examples of the increasing resistance as strength increases, see the various workout plans and exercises in the back of this book.

If proper form in any given exercise or sport is difficult for you to understand or achieve, reach out to fitness experts and find the resources required to do the exercise right. Because without exercising the right way, you will mistake activity for accomplishment and your fitness goals will stay an arm's length away.

After multiple golf lessons, Tom admitted that while his overall game had improved, the strides were slow going. Yet every time he approached the ball, he no longer thought about trying to become the next Tiger Woods. He thought about his grip, his hips, and his follow-through. He ensured he used the same precision every time. He'd become a proper-form nut. And the results were slowly taking hold.

Every single time we get the opportunity to exercise, we have the ability either to do it right, or to just be satisfied that we're doing it at all. The question is, do you want to be the person who exercises, or the person who's fit? The difference is all in the form.

New Year / New Me

I've always had mixed emotions about New Year's Day. On one hand, the number of personal training clients always increases. A vast number of individuals decide (year after year) that January 1 will be the kickoff to better fitness. On the other hand, the fitness nut inside me dislikes it greatly. The days, weeks, and months after the New Year make exercising at the gym nearly overwhelming. Almost all equipment is in use, poor exercise form is rampant, and there's an air of annoyance from the gym regulars. We all wait for the end of February to come so that the crowds will subside.

That's the routine I saw. Each year, people would make a New Year's resolution to get fit and would show tremendous drive for a couple of months. When the new program became difficult to maintain, or the results didn't come fast enough, the newest members of the gym would disappear. Once April or May hit, gym participation was back to "normal" levels.

As a fitness-obsessed personal trainer, I thought I understood what was happening. People didn't have a game plan, or the proper support to make a long-lasting commitment. And when push came to shove, they didn't have the strength to stay the course.

As an overweight and purposefully lazy person, I realized that I'd been wrong. I had spent more time in gyms by the age of 30 than most people would in their entire lifetimes, but now I was scared to go back and face the judgment and physical difficulties.

I struggled through my workouts, and the soreness and lack of energy made the couch look all the more inviting.

Scarier still, specific routines and workouts that used to be the foundation of my fitness nirvana were now difficult and unsettling.

Yet I went to the gym every day, because I had to. I knew that my nutritional changes had started to reap benefits, but true health could not be found only in a proper diet. My body needed physical activity; it needed to be challenged.

I also had to learn that I had different limits now than I had when I was fit. Back then, the idea of struggling to do a push-up would have been laughable. Now, my arms would shake violently, and the sensation of my stomach hitting the floor was uncomfortable. It would have been easy to push the gas, though, and to make myself hate the pain (or worse, the failure).

As difficult as it was, I had to learn to balance myself. It was the physical activity that was important, not the level of push-up being performed. I dropped to my knees so that I could continue my workout with proper form. As days turned into weeks, and weeks into months, the pain and soreness began to subside. I started enjoying working out again, as I could sense that my body was starting to depend on the exertion once again. And it was encouraging to see the progress in my strength and conditioning.

Getting tremendously out of shape on my journey from Fit2Fat helped me realize just how hard getting into shape is when you're nowhere close. Until this journey, I was always in great shape and very active. This weight-gain process helped put into perspective the journey back to physical fitness. My old routines didn't work. My gym ego had taken a beating. Strength and conditioning take effort to maintain; they are surprisingly fleeting if we're not careful.

In the end, the most critical lesson I learned is that the only true path to fitness is that of balance. We must find balance in our lives to make time for our bodies. We must find balance at the gym to make certain that we don't lose interest and so that we continue to see results. And we must find balance in our form and our approach to the exercises themselves.

In other words, torture through excessive pain or through boredom is not the answer. It's about making a choice to become fit and then taking it one day at a time. My friend's payback smile was the first reminder of many that my journey back to fit was going to be challenging. But with every challenge in our lives, the rewards soon speak for themselves. My motivation never waned—well, not for more than a moment—though I was forced to take a new and more measured approach. I soon found that with my consistent nutritional plan, the results continued to mount in my second and third months of Fat2Fit. After the first month of weight loss, which was extreme, the weight loss started to fall into a more consistent pattern.

In month two, I dropped another 12 pounds. In month three, I lost over nine. While the days of losing 19 pounds in four weeks were gone, the fact that I was still losing weight was encouraging. It's easy to get excited about the sheer volume of weight loss early on, and about the final pounds that are lost when you reach a goal.

It's the middle pounds that are tough. At that point you're still struggling with obesity but starting to understand what it's like to feel healthy. Once those middle pounds start to fade, with progress slowing, the journey to becoming fit gets more difficult. We realize, as 10, then 20, then 30 pounds have been shed, that we'll need something beyond the right nutrition or fitness plan.

For all of the spinach shakes, push-ups, fully prepared meals, and pull-ups, there's one final ingredient that's critical for any turnaround from Fat2Fit to be long-lasting. Surprisingly, it has nothing to do with the person who is overweight. It has everything to do with those around him or her.

Because taking control of your health is not a journey that can be undertaken alone.

CHAPTER 7

KICKING AND SCREAMING TO THE TOP OF THE MOUNTAIN

I didn't want to do it. It was too soon, too much, and too scary. Even worse, I felt guilted into it, and I wasn't sure that any number of excuses would get me out of the activity he had planned for me.

This was supposed to be a relaxing long weekend. I didn't have to work, it was the middle of the holiday season, and my brother Erik was in town. Besides, I was experiencing something I'd never experienced before becoming overweight—the complete desire *not* to work out.

As you know by now, working out used to be my drug, my addiction. I couldn't get enough of it. In fact, I found myself going through withdrawal if I hadn't been to the gym in a couple days. But after seven months of being sedentary, I'd gotten used to long afternoons in front of the television.

I'd assumed that my brother's visit was going to be low-key. He knew what shape I was in, and this was the holiday season, after all. I should have known better. Erik was a tremendous influence on me as I grew up. He was just as active as I was, if not more so (which helps explain my original interest). And he hadn't gone through seven months of rest and relaxation; he was still fit, and no amount of extra weight on me was going to stop him from a brotherly tradition.

Exercise was how we bonded. Every visit was filled with hikes, exercise routines, runs, and the like. Erik tried to push me to new heights, even when I was fit. It was a tradition—and it was going to stay a tradition, in spite of my changed attitude toward exercise.

When Erik sat down to talk to me about our "activity," he seemed to sense my trepidation. Before I could spit out a single excuse as to why we should take it easy, he laid out an aggressive hike that would have pushed me when I was healthy. This wasn't going to be pretty.

I took the necessary precautions, loading myself up with so much water you'd have thought I was a newly graduated Boy Scout, and gave my wife an extra hug in case the wilderness got the best of me. Then off my brother and I went for a hike.

It took only 15 minutes before I started getting winded. That would have been the perfect moment to turn around and head back down the mountain. But my brother knew me (and what my body needed) better than I did. So he kept walking. He stayed slightly ahead of me, forcing me to keep up and not get too far behind. When I took extended water breaks, he'd push me to go a little farther up the trail.

My body was revolting: my legs were burning, my lungs felt as if they were going to explode, and I could already feel the soreness my body would punish me with the next day.

But the physical pain was nothing compared to how my mind felt. I had unnatural thoughts about hurting my brother and crazy ideas about how to force him to end the hike. I also considered numerous excuses, each a little more far-fetched than the last, to manipulate him into taking it easy. In the end, though, the best I could muster was to play on his sympathies, talking about how trying the journey was and the tremendous toll it was taking on my physical and mental health.

And yet . . . we continued up the trail. Erik toyed with my emotions by repeatedly telling me we were going to go only a bit farther, only to let minutes pass before he spoke again. But still I followed him.

By the time my brother stopped and turned around, I was profusely sweating, and my legs felt like jelly. I hadn't fully caught my breath since the bottom of the trail, and I wasn't sure I could make it back to our car. Then I looked around and realized just how far we had walked—and it was a long way. I had accomplished this; I had hiked farther than I could have hoped for, given my unfit state, and I felt an enormous amount of pride.

As my brother passed by me and started the trek back, I loyally followed him downhill. On my way down, something struck me: I hadn't gotten myself up the mountain at all. If I'd had my way, I would still be lying on the couch, working only my finger muscles as I channel-surfed.

My brother had pushed me into action, gently but determinedly forcing me out of my comfort zone. It was a strange feeling. In the past, I'd always been up for a challenge—the harder the better. But for one of the first times in my life, I would have chosen to do nothing on this day. And yet I did something—more than I would have thought possible. But only because someone knew what I needed more than I did. And that someone made sure I got it—in spite of myself.

The Biggest Winner

There's no rulebook for personal training. To the best of my knowledge, no author has penned *Personal Training for Dummies*. Sure, there are classes and certifications, primarily focused around providing proper instruction, technique, and safety.

But taking on the mental and emotional challenges of a client is not something to be found in a certification. Not because those challenges aren't important, but because they're hard to quantify and even harder to manage. And yet, above all other characteristics, a personal trainer's approach to the emotional/mental aspect of fitness is what distinguishes one of us from another.

You have the screamers—militant personal trainers who believe they can scare any individual into proper fitness (and probably scare the actual weight off in the process). In shouting their commands, they generate a sore throat, concerned stares of passersby, and genuine fear in their clientele.

On the other end of the spectrum you have the healers—the walking version of *Chicken Soup for the Soul*. These trainers utter encouraging words of support, along with inspirational slogans and stories to stir the deepest motivation in their trainees.

I took a different approach—I was the jack of all trades. I tried almost everything under the sun to get my clients to reach their fitness goals. While I never resorted to out-and-out screaming or to visualizations, I *did* use a vast array of weapons to get my clients to take necessary steps for their own health.

If particular clients were down on themselves, I would try to pick them up through encouragement. I'd tell them that I believed in them, and that they could accomplish anything they put their mind to. If they were feeling lazy or not engaged, I would challenge their commitment to the cause, explaining that only they could truly change their lifestyle. I would be excited when they accomplished even the smallest of sets, hoping that they'd be encouraged and motivated to continue. When that didn't work, I would try guilt. And if that failed too, I'd feign exasperation (or let my real exasperation show).

No matter how many tactics I used, the results were spotty at best. Some clients listened for a while, but even they lost my message as time wore on. Others seemed impervious to my every approach, suspiciously countering any new tactic I tried to employ.

Yet after I gained 70-plus pounds, I realized exactly what the problem had been. I had come to believe, in the old days, that I just hadn't found the right "message" that would speak to my clients. I stubbornly believed that my own breakthrough as a personal trainer was just one more training session away. I was going to find the magic formula.

Well, I was wrong. The epiphany was not just a session away. Personal trainers can be a lot of things, but they're only one piece of the puzzle. And not the most important piece either. To truly change your approach to health, a support network is essential.

As I said before, when I was fit I believed that a person who is overweight simply needed to decide to get in shape and the rest would fall into place.

When I was unfit and working toward becoming healthy, I woke up every day doubting what I could accomplish and trying my best to do as little as I could. I knew what my goals were, because I had mapped them out. I also had the knowledge and know-how to reach those goals. And yet it was a struggle every day.

In fact, if left to my own devices, I'd have made more wrong decisions than right ones. I'd have rationalized that an extra day off wouldn't be a problem. I'd have become my own worst enemy (and at times I was) in my fight to become fit.

Taking control of your health is quite literally a fight for your life. Now, having experienced being overweight firsthand, I understand both the importance and the difficulty of that fight. Your mind and body work against you every day, making what should be simple decisions very difficult, and enticing you with quick fixes, lazy days, and unhealthy choices that feel a little too easy to make.

It's in those dark moments of choice that a strong, established support network is vital. The support group can be made up of one or many. They can be family, friends, or a mix of both. But they have to be individuals who provide you with two things that you won't be able to provide yourself consistently every single day of the journey to becoming healthy—honesty and belief. And more importantly, they must be intimately involved in your journey; they have to know when you're struggling or need a dose of honesty or encouragement, sometimes even before you realize you need it.

This support network requires two parts in order to develop into the final key of your success; one comes from them, the other comes from you.

Yin and Yang

Prior to the birth of our first child, Lynn and I had extensive conversations about the type of parents we would be. We openly wondered which of us would be the disciplinarian, laying down the law at any given moment. Which one would melt like a Popsicle in the summer when our kids flashed their "puppy dog eyes" at us? And who would be the brave soul able to stomach the nightmares, colds, and flus that were sure to greet us?

When I was growing up, my mom and dad fell into different roles. I adjusted to those roles and knew who to go to, and for what reason.

Mom was there for the "softer" stuff—whether it be a hug, taking care of a scraped knee, or offering a cold cloth in the midst of a bout of stomach flu. Mom knew how to care, and how to make sure that we had everything we needed when things weren't going well. And she believed in and encouraged me, even when I was full of self-doubt.

Dad, on the other hand, was the pusher. He drove me to do more and to be more. He made sure that I was pushing myself in my sports and activities of choice, with a slightly stern approach. Yet his prodding made me try a little harder to reach my own goals.

He was also the disciplinarian. I wouldn't have been fearful of bringing home a poor report card with less than glowing marks to Mom. She would probably have gotten me a snack and told me to try a bit harder. Dad, on the other hand, kept me on the straight and narrow. He pushed when he needed to, and made me see the consequences of my actions. Tough love was a necessity, helping me to see the "reality" of the world and make appropriate decisions.

In truth, I so eagerly talked to Lynn about the various roles we would fill for our own children because I realized how important the balance that I'd had was. I'd had a yin and a yang growing up: I was in constant balance between someone padding the corners and someone else pushing me into them so that I'd learn to avoid them for myself. For my own children, I was anxious to keep that balance, even if it meant that Lynn would inherit the role of disciplinarian and I would be there with the princess Band-Aids.

Whether we're small children, unruly teenagers, confused young adults, or busy and distracted adults, something inside of us craves balance. Needing both sides of the equation, we tend to shy away from extremes.

So why should our approach to health and fitness be any different? Our bodies and minds react poorly to diets and exercise routines that require unsettling extremes. We search instead for options that balance our need to be healthy with our busy lives and time constraints.

We want great nutrition but don't want to break the bank to achieve it. We want healthy meals without having to cut our work down to part-time to find the time to prepare them. In other words, balance is essential.

Yet too often we approach a new nutritional goal or exercise routine out of balance. Taking a radical approach is a risk. Not only do we quickly realize that a three-hour lentil dish isn't feasible on a Wednesday night or that 90 minutes of cardio kickboxing is ill-advised (for both time and health reasons), but it becomes painfully obvious that our unbalanced approach isn't sustainable for the long haul. This is not to say that we shouldn't push ourselves. We should. But it's critical to realize that our chances of success are much greater when we have the necessary support. Part of balance is realizing that alone we're vulnerable; we need those around us to rally, encourage, and catch us before we spin too far in any one direction. We need our yin and our yang—our encouragement and our accountability.

The journey to fitness is one of self-doubt. Every day you're confronted with images of individuals in better shape and in better control of their own health. You come face to face with bad habits, strange cravings, and newly discovered weak areas. You're constantly reminded of how you ended up in your current state, and how quickly you could fall back into the same destructive patterns.

There will be moments when you don't believe it's possible to accomplish everything you set out to do. It's in those moments—the ones when you physically, mentally, or emotionally feel yourself failing—that you need a yin, an encourager.

That's not to say that you need an enabler—someone who's going to excuse you for breaking down too often in your meal plans, or skipping a week's worth of exercising. My parents, no matter how encouraging, never gave us the option of giving up or failing—they just made it easier to succeed.

An encourager will be there to listen on the difficult days and to remind you why you're on the journey in the first place. If the lentil dinner is making you rethink your new nutrition plan or the cardio workout led to a minor injury, the encourager will be entrenched in the journey with you, willing you to push through one more day or to prepare another week's worth of meals (or even to steer you away from the processed foods in the grocery store).

The encourager also knows your weak points and understands the emotional and mental struggle that being overweight (and trying to become fit) encompasses. He or she sees where you're slipping before you do and can give a supportive nudge to get you back on track.

But too much encouragement can be a problem in the journey back to health—because, as human beings, we know how to push the buttons of the encourager and to play on his or her sympathies when we're at our lowest. Hence the need of a yang, and with it the accountability.

For as much as we need to be understood as we fight for our health, we sometimes need a kick in the pants. We fall into ruts, or accept that it's okay to take a day off from the gym or have a cheat day with fast food. At those moments no amount of simple encouragement will get us back on track. We need tough love.

The disciplinarians in your life will provide you with a dose of honesty that you desperately need. No, they won't push it so far as to become demotivators, but they'll remind you of why you're on the journey and point out that you're not going to reach your goals without hard work.

Disciplinarians pull you off the couch and to the gym when you really want to stay home, and they keep you from the fast-food restaurant when a Happy Meal seems to be the only worthwhile goal in life. In short, they don't accept your excuses and don't let you keep yourself from success. They will you to succeed when it's easiest to give up.

Interestingly, both roles have one thing in common: they push you forward. A support team to better health has nothing to do with excusing poor choices, applauding a break in your exercise routine, or telling you that "no one will know" if you cheat. That's not support; it's a one-way ticket back to your old ways and waistline.

The true yin and yang of support provide encouragement and discipline in equal parts, and both keep you on track toward your goals. Like the balance you require in your workouts, you need balance in your support network to truly change your lifestyle.

The yin and the yang you need are usually already right there in your life, champing at the bit to help. I encourage you to look around and share your goals with people you know. You might be surprised at how easily a team forms. However, the support team is only half the equation. The other half may be most important (and courageous of all). And it comes from you.

The Public Declaration

There were certain subjects in school that were clearly not my strengths. While I seemed to excel at gym, trudging into social studies wasn't the favorite part of my day. That's not to say I was the stereotypical meathead football player. I was just a bit more selective in the classes and subjects that held my attention.

Attention wasn't a problem in history classes; I enjoyed them and was fascinated by stories in which the fates of many were decided by the words and actions of a few. Like everyone else, I was taught about some of the most impactful individuals in history—world leaders, inventors, military generals, and presidents. While he was before my time, I was fascinated by the words and actions of one such man—John F. Kennedy.

Kennedy was a unique individual in that he could eloquently move a nation with words of encouragement, driving individuals into action through a single speech. He is rightfully famous for the "Ask not what your country can do for you" line in his inauguration speech in 1961.

But Kennedy gave another speech to a joint session of Congress in May 1961 that would prove the power of publicly declaring a goal and commitment, no matter how far-fetched or impossible it seemed.

When Kennedy spoke to Congress on that occasion, the subject of his speech (space exploration) was an audacious idea. While the United States was deep in an arms race with the Soviet Union, the idea of exploring the reaches of space seemed far-fetched and a bit crazy.

President Kennedy could have stood in front of the room and asked for minor advances in the space program. He could have stated a long-term goal to reach space long after his presidency had ended. Instead, he took an altogether riskier and much-critiqued approach. He (literally) reached for the stars.

Kennedy challenged NASA and the United States to put a man on the moon by the end of the decade. For many, the idea was laughable and impossible. For Kennedy, it was a mandate.

Two and a half years later, John F. Kennedy was assassinated. Yet, shockingly, just over eight years later (and six months before the end of the decade), NASA's Apollo 11 mission would land the first humans on the moon.

Historians alike would rightfully credit the proper funding, political support, and expertise of NASA for accomplishing such an impossible feat in such an impossible amount of time. But the true key to making this happen was the fact that Kennedy made a public declaration, in effect challenging himself and those around him to find a way to make it happen, rather than focus on why it couldn't be done.

The point of the story is that a public declaration is a vital (and perhaps the most important) part of attaining our goals, regardless of the scope. That applies to us as individuals, too.

Every single day, millions of Americans want to change their lifestyle. They want to be healthier, find fitness, and make an impact on their medical well-being. But too often they do so alone, and in silence. They take the approach that it's better to keep their goal quiet until they have succeeded. The reality, though, is that we keep our goals and commitments to ourselves for two reasons: fear of critique and fear of accountability.

It's easy to feel like we live in a cruel world—one that may be more interested in knocking us down to size than in lifting us up. Therefore, the thought of publicly declaring fitness and health goals is intimidating. We fear that such a declaration will invite criticism, disbelief, and discouragement.

In addition, publicly sharing goals and commitment inspires another fear—that of accountability. When we're at home alone and fall off the nutritional wagon or skip a workout, we're the only ones who know it. It's our little secret. But make your goals known, and you're suddenly surrounded by people who will notice your poor choices or lack of effort.

By publicly declaring your journey, you essentially close off the escape route. You're no longer the only one who will know if you fail. And while disappointing ourselves can take a toll, disappointing others is much more difficult. We suddenly become accountable for our actions.

Trust me, you'll be surprised at how quickly the excuses go away once you've stated your intentions. You're now accountable, and you know it.

No matter how many meal plans, exercises, and recipes are provided, the spark to change has to come from within the individual. There comes a time, perhaps after years of dithering, when you make the decision that you're ready for change and want to take the necessary steps to turn things around.

That's the time to publicly declare your intentions. Such a declaration is the first step toward making a permanent and long-lasting commitment to health. We need as many people as possible to hold us accountable to the life change we so clearly desire for ourselves. We need to ask for those aforementioned two things that we won't consistently be able to provide ourselves throughout the journey: honesty and belief.

That's not to say that every single person wanting to make a health change needs to start a blog or write a letter to Oprah. For some, a public declaration may be made only to a spouse, a friend, or a coworker. But the words, the desires, and the overall goals need to be shared and spoken. Only then can true accomplishment be achieved.

Part of the reason for a declaration's importance is what it signifies: such a bold, public commitment can be made only by an individual convinced that the end result is a given—it's not a question of *if* it can be accomplished, but merely a question of *how* and *by when*. If your goals and desires for a better you are kept to yourself, you'll live in a world of "I can't do this." The moment you make those goals known, you force yourself to live in a world of "How can I do this?" And you find a way.

Moreover, you're no longer alone. The moment you share your aspirations for your own health and fitness, you invite your support group to start building around you. The team and the declaration go hand in hand. You can't have one without the other. And both will propel you on your journey to health.

My public declaration was a little different than most, given my goals and journey. It went out quietly enough, but soon I got more feedback than I could have ever expected. Fortunately, every negative tweet or e-mail came with several encouraging ones. My wife and a few friends made for an incredible support team from the get-go, but I soon realized that my support team extended beyond my immediate circle. The online community was there to encourage me and hold me accountable. I was motivated beyond anything I've ever experienced before.

In 1961, long before the world was ready for it, one man publicly declared that the United States would accomplish something never done before—land a human on the moon—and would do so in a timeframe so audacious that few believed it was possible.

Eight-plus years later, the goal was accomplished. Not just because people worked hard and NASA had enough resources to make it happen, but because one person found the bravery to make the declaration, inviting criticism and accountability—and, most importantly, issuing an unwavering mandate to ensure that the goal was accomplished.

True health doesn't take place in the kitchen or at the gym. The path to health comes from announcing your intentions out loud and working with those who are there to help you meet your goals and fulfill your mandate.

The next fad diet or fitness regime will be an extreme, for sure. They almost always are. Diet and weight-loss plans focus on what you're eating, with exercise viewed as a bonus to the food restrictions. Fitness plans, on the other hand, put their focus in the gym or workout room. Results come from "sweating it out," and diet or nutritional guidelines are added on as friendly reminders to maximize results by eating the right things.

These approaches are not the answer. As I learned from this journey, balance is the key. Proper nutrition is as essential to significant weight loss as maintaining a consistent workout routine.

But we can't stop there. Achieving our goals requires a balanced approach that is sustainable because we have made a public declaration and have a support team to help us on our way.

The proper nutritional, fitness, and support guidelines positioned me as I worked my way back toward being fit. As the months went by, I continued to lose weight toward my goals.

Yet I was about to face an unspoken barrier to reaching fitness and health goals. It's the dreaded "final 15 pounds"—and to date, it's the true "wall" that everyone hits. It's also the one subject no one seems to want to confront.

Until now.

CHAPTER 8

THE LAST 15 POUNDS

Caught off guard by a brand-new emotion, I positioned my feet just in front of the scale. I was hesitant to step on. This wasn't a big deal, right? I had gone through this same routine every single Saturday morning for over 10 months. Why should today be any different?

As I looked down at the scale, the feeling of trepidation increased. Taking a deep breath, I stepped on, staring forward rather than down. The results of the last two weeks had not gone according to plan, and I was afraid that today's results would be no better.

Just two weeks earlier, I had stepped on the scale to see another few pounds lost from my once-overweight frame. I was close, so close, to reaching my goal. I knew that at this stage in the process every pound mattered. I was thrilled and proud that I had lost more weight in just a week.

I literally hopped off the scale that day, excited to do more. I devoured my spinach shake, prepared a nutritious lunch, and started reviewing my workout routine for the day. I was in the zone. I didn't have to think as much about eating nutritiously anymore. And my body had once again started to crave the workouts. At last, I was starting to feel like myself!

Later that day, I conquered the grocery store with ease. Sure, I had twinges of longing at the ice-cold display of Mountain Dew, but the bottled water I carried with me quickly quelled them. I stayed on the outside aisles of the store, loading my cart with vegetables, fruits, and lean meats.

It felt great to be over the hump. I didn't find myself as tempted to eat fast food (either that or my cravings had just become easier to control!), and my biweekly preparation of meals was now such a part of our family routine that my wife and I split duties, surprising each other with the recipe we'd chosen for the coming days.

And the workouts—oh, the workouts! Draining, exhausting, but addicting. I once again found myself actively looking forward to my trips to the gym. Most important, I was more comfortable in my own skin. I knew that I was far from done, but it was great to be feeling like myself again.

One week later, I jumped onto the scale eagerly. I was certain that more pounds had been shed, and I would be one step closer to my prejourney weight.

My first thought as the number registered: the scale had to be running out of juice. It was impossible that I had lost so little. I had such higher expectations for my progress. I stepped off, readjusted my weight (as if this would help), and tried again. Not surprisingly, the number on the scale hadn't changed. I stepped off yet again, picked up the scale, and shook it. Maybe it wasn't properly calibrated.

This lasted for three more minutes—up, off, shake—until I finally realized that there would be no difference in my weight no matter how many times I got on and off the scale. I exhaled, considered the big picture, and found renewed determination to work harder and follow my workout routines with even greater care.

That evening, Lynn asked if I'd be interested in going out to dinner, given that it had been so long since we'd had a real date. I declined, explaining that I didn't want any extra calories and needed to make sure I ate as nutritiously as possible. (For the record, I did not win Husband of the Week.)

I put in an extra-long workout the next day and, while shopping, traversed the grocery store with such gusto that I'm sure store employees and shoppers were slightly alarmed. I became militant about what went into my cart, sensing that a few more fruits and vegetables would do the trick.

I personally prepared all of the meals for the week, playing it off to my wife that I wanted her to have a break. In truth, I had to make sure the meals were perfectly prepared. And I drank more water than usual each day, just to help things along.

A few exhausting and difficult days later, I found myself hesitant to get on the scale. What if I hadn't lost enough weight? What if the weeks of dropping multiple pounds were over? Even more concerning, what if my workout routines and nutritional guidelines weren't producing the results I had expected them to?

My final comforting thought was that I had followed all of my meal plans, hadn't allowed myself any splurges, and had completed my workouts with more ease than I had at any point in the last four months.

Okay, the moment of truth. I stepped up on the scale and glanced down. I blinked. If I thought last week was bad, I wasn't prepared for this week's scale surprise.

One week was bad enough, but another week of inadequate weight loss? After *that* week of dedicated exercise and nutrition? How was that even possible?

It's About the Journey, Not the Destination

Michael Jordan is the icon of professional basketball, the standard by which all current and future players are judged. When one thinks of Jordan, many thoughts come to mind—his redefining of the sport, his six championships, and his ability to perform superhuman acts on the court. There's no denying his excellence and the consistent "product" he displayed in every game.

Yet that Michael Jordan—the one that stays with us—wasn't always viewed in that way. In fact, years before, his critics wondered if he'd ever live up to his billing and accomplish what the greats had: win a championship.

Michael Jordan came into the National Basketball Association as a phenom. He had led his college team (North Carolina) to a national championship, and it was assumed that his abilities would translate to the professional ranks. Yet three years into his career, Jordan had a critic for every fan, questioning his ability to be a team player, to make those around him better, and to be a proper defender.

It was painfully obvious that he was trying to do too much. His team, the Chicago Bulls, kept having mediocre records and losing in the first round of the playoffs. The pressure and desire to achieve a championship was taking its toll on Jordan and his fans. Jordan simply wasn't improving. In fact, the more he tried to do, the less he seemed to accomplish.

So Michael Jordan went back to square one. He started working with a fitness trainer who helped him build a stronger core and greater endurance. He practiced incessantly in the gym, trying to perfect his technique and build further basketball skills. He worked tirelessly on his defensive game.

Even with that dedication, progress in his overall goals came at a slow pace. Years after being called a lazy defender, more concerned with scoring points, Jordan won his first Defensive Player of the Year award. His Bulls got better as well, advancing out of the first round of the playoffs, and started to knock on the door of a berth in the NBA Finals.

Yet Jordan again hit a wall. For as good as he and his team had become, the Bulls continued to lose to a better team each year—the Detroit Pistons. Again at a crossroads, Jordan had another choice. He could continue to press, sure that he would win a championship, or he could question his current status and figure out how to improve.

Jordan studied one nemesis on the Pistons, Joe Dumars. In spite of Jordan's better natural talent, when the Bulls and Pistons reached the sixth or seventh game of their annual series, Dumars and the Pistons seemed to have a bit more in the tank.

So Jordan developed a morning workout group to get better and gain further endurance through the long NBA season. As Jordan committed to the extra workouts, teammates followed suit. Together, the team's chemistry and endurance grew.

In the 1990–1991 season, Michael Jordan finally broke through and carried the Chicago Bulls to the NBA Finals. That same year, the Bulls won the first of what would be six championship titles with Jordan at the helm.

It would have been easy to start to relax/coast. Yet Jordan's morning workouts continued. More teammates joined the program. And he was the first one in the gym and the last one to leave. In the end, Jordan faced this choice: to focus on the destination or to focus on the journey (believing that the destination was a given). He chose the latter.

As we approach our own health and fitness goals, it's easy to get lost in the destination. We pinpoint a weight, a dress size, or a waist measurement which will signify that we've accomplished everything we hoped for. That numerical goal becomes the be-all and end-all. In other words, we ignore Jordan's model and become obsessed over whether we reached a certain number.

When we're overweight and decide to become healthy, our initial positive changes in nutrition and fitness have an immediate impact on our measurements and weight. Pounds come off in droves, and we drop pants sizes so quickly it's hard to find a pair that comfortably fits.

All the nutrition and fitness plans we follow tell us to stay the course and our goals will be met. In most cases, everything seems to progress. That is, until we plateau. This leveling off happens even when we remain committed to our nutrition and our workouts. Despite our best efforts, the pounds stop dropping off. The pants we now fit into stay around a month longer than we had hoped.

Of course we get frustrated. Thus begins a cycle in which all decisions and actions around our health are based on measurements or numbers on a scale. If we drop a pound, it all seems worth it and we celebrate. If we gain a pound or simply maintain, we become depressed, or worse, convinced that something is flawed with our approach and that all the hard work isn't worth it.

Despite the universality of this issue, the nutrition and fitness routines out there tend to avoid talk of the "final 15 pounds." It's the unspoken problem with losing weight: a plateau will come—it's inevitable—and most of us are left feeling helpless and alone in the face of it.

Well, here's what I learned the hard way. The final 10 to 15 pounds comprise a mental battle as much as a physical one. And in order to overcome the mental and physical rigors, we must change the game. We must forget about the numbers.

True health does not dictate that you weigh a certain amount or have a waist of a certain number of inches. Health is a state of being. It's about making the right decisions every single day.

While true, that understanding of the bigger picture doesn't make the frustration of the final 15 pounds any less difficult to deal with. But if we're to push through and achieve the change we're looking for, we need to keep looking at this bigger picture. We can't continue to improve by narrowing our focus down to numbers and results. If we do, our ultimate destination (which has nothing to do with a specific number) will remain out of reach.

Here's what I learned the hard way. The final 10 to 15 pounds comprise a mental battle as much as a physical one. And in order to overcome the mental and physical rigors, we must forget about the numbers.

When we reach the final 15 pounds, we're at the same crossroads that Michael Jordan faced in his early and middle career. The more he pressed to reach his destination, the less likely it seemed he would achieve it. But when he stepped back and focused on the choices and impacts he was making on his overall journey, Jordan was able to excel at the highest level for years.

The key to tackling the last 15 pounds isn't to become obsessed with a scale or a tape measure. It's to reflect on how our goals fit into our lifestyle. We need to find ways—large and small—to make our approach to weight loss part of our everyday life. Becoming healthy isn't something we can compartmentalize into a "45-minute" workout. Our decisions about health will affect all aspects of our daily life. We need to accept that losing weight isn't just about restrictive diets or obsessive workouts; it's about making the right choices every day and believing that these choices will make us happy and keep us healthy well beyond the program's or plan's intended time limits.

Changing the Game

We all seem to have a roadmap for what adulthood will bring us. Although the actual map differs for each person, there's a typically prescriptive path that everyone expects to follow.

After high school, we have to make the decision whether to go through at least four more years of education or immediately enter the workforce. Concurrently or soon after, we face the freedom of moving out of our parents' house, getting our first "real" job, and starting to build our own lives.

Next comes serious dating (beyond the more superficial experiences of romance) and trying to find a significant other to spend a lifetime with (or, in my case, someone who will put up with you!), followed by marriage and potentially children.

No matter how you get to this stage in life, most individuals share another common goal: becoming a homeowner. After a few years of living in apartments, dealing with loud neighbors above and below you, rising rent costs, and the realization that you're not building any sort of equity, you find the idea of owning a home increasingly attractive.

Typically, this first major purchase is called a starter home. It qualifies as an actual home in that you inherit a mortgage and can (and do!) nail anything to the wall that you'd like without incurring a hit on a security deposit. But the starter home isn't designed as a long-term fit. There are a limited number of bedrooms and an even more limited number of bathrooms. You're lucky if the kitchen can fit more than one person comfortably, storage space is nonexistent, and the idea of expansion is simply audacious. But for the current situation, it's perfect.

And then things start to change. You begin collecting belongings throughout the years—tokens and trinkets and furniture that you can't bear to relinquish. Children often enter the equation, first taking over any spare bedrooms and then taking control of half of every bathroom.

With drawers and closets filled to capacity with toys, books, and puzzles, you start looking for creative places to use as storage. And trying to feed a group of people in the kitchen now is laughable—it's easier to put out some television trays than deal with a full-fledged dining room table.

Finally you wake up one day and feel like your house is going to explode. There's no room for anything, and you realize that either the family and possessions have to stop growing (in fact, have to shrink!) or you're going to need a bigger house. Simply put, the starter home has served its purpose. You've reached the ceiling (both literally and figuratively).

As a result, and if you're fortunate, you upgrade. You sell the starter home (likely to another up-and-coming couple) and move into a home with actual storage, more than two bedrooms, and enough bathrooms that the children have one "just for them." You ensure that every room has closet space and that there's potential for expansion. You're now able to increase your family and/or possessions to the next level.

Perhaps it's the reality of a starter home's limitations that makes us realize the routines of the past don't work in the present. When we see overflowing closets, we know it's time for more storage.

Being overweight is like the good old days when you were still living with your parents. You didn't worry about space back then, and you worried less about having the basic necessities around you. Similarly, as a person who is overweight with no goal to be fit, you eat what you want, when you want, and any physical exertion is on your terms alone.

When you make the decision to lose weight and get healthy, you realize it's time to move out and buy your own starter home, as it were. Your starter home, which is small and manageable, offers a level of control you aren't used to.

And it works for you. The starter home of health and fitness is about balance, choice, and persistence. Your meals are prepared and measured according to plan, and you focus on following demanding workout routines to get the results you need.

Yet all too often, as we've seen, the results start to slow down. You aren't getting the drop in pounds or inches that you're used to, and you aren't sure why. The answer might surprise you.

When our bodies start to get healthy, they require change. People are often surprised to learn that I needed a 3,000-calorie diet to maintain my pre–weight gain body. Why? Because when the body is operating at its optimum level, considerable energy is required. It takes plenty of fuel for the body to continue to lose fat and build muscle. In essence, your body needs more to do more.

When we're nearing our health goals, our bodies start to require more nutrients and activity to maintain performance. If we don't change (that is, if we stay in our starter home), we can only go so far—there's a ceiling that we will hit, and the results will crawl to a halt.

We're smart enough as homeowners to know when it's time to leave the starter home behind and upgrade to a larger space. When we reach the ceiling in our own health, we're not so savvy. Typically, we either quit or go more extreme with the restrictions. We believe that if we cut a few more calories out of our diet the weight will start to come off again, but the opposite is actually true.

If the body starts to require more energy, but isn't getting it, it goes into "retention mode." It holds on to fat and the limited amount of nutrients it's getting, just to maintain its current state. The body won't continue to become leaner because there's simply not enough fuel to do so.

One of the hardest lessons to learn is that when we reach our health plateau, we need to move out of the starter home and into a larger space. Many times, we need to actually increase our caloric intake (still with healthy choices!) as we continue to advance in our physical activity. However we do it, we must *adjust*.

The human body is amazing in that it offers clues as to when a systemic change is required in our diet and/or fitness routine: it stops making progress. You can either continue to push against the ceiling, becoming frustrated that no results are coming, or you can upgrade your diet and make sure that your body has enough fuel and energy to continue to shed weight and build lean muscle.

When you're progressing through your life roadmap, moving from a starter home to the house you'll live in for

30 years is a momentous occasion. For many, it means you've arrived. The plateau in your own health is equally momentous. Finally, your body is starting to perform at a level it's never seen before.

By stepping back and seeing the big picture, you can make the necessary adjustment to exit the plateau. The next step is to recognize that it's time to move into a larger space, as it were—more calories of healthy foods and a higher level of physical activity. With that adjustment, suddenly the plateau disappears, and the weight again starts to drop off.

One Degree of Separation

First as a personal trainer, and then more intimately as I became overweight, I have been surprised that we treat our own health as if we need only a high school diploma to survive. We learn the basics, perfect the basics, and continue to do the basics . . . over and over and over. We never advance. We never push ourselves.

When we're overweight, even the idea of physical activity is scary, exhausting, and painful. Just walking into the gym can be tiring, and getting onto a treadmill and walking for a few minutes is enough to send even the strongest-willed person home, defeated.

Yet every time we get on the wagon (or treadmill), we get stronger. Our bodies start to learn how to operate better. The weight begins to come off. For the first time, we start to feel what "healthy" means.

So we take baby steps forward. Instead of simply strolling on the treadmill, we walk briskly. We increase the weights we're using. We add additional resistance to the elliptical machine. Before we know it, we've lost almost unfathomable amounts of weight, and we feel great. As we approach our overall goals, we can power through any workout routine that we're faced with.

At the gym, we start to identify with those others who are there day in and day out, as opposed to the new member struggling in the corner. We actually enjoy our workouts and are more and more impressed with the fact that we can run a 5K without collapsing, or that we get through an exercise class with the best form of the bunch.

And then we plateau. The weight loss stops. The inches remain. We're so close to our end goals, and yet so far from where we want to be. We agonize over this, but we don't truly change anything where it matters most—in our workouts.

Once we reach an acceptable level of performance, we revel in the high output and increased energy. We don't feel sore anymore, and we attribute that to better health as opposed to not working hard enough. We convince ourselves that a healthy person wouldn't be exhausted or sore through a workout. The lack of pain is our reward for all the earlier horrific workouts that made every small movement the next day feel like agony.

Yet the only way to overcome the plateau and achieve long-lasting results is to continue to add to our workouts, change our routines, and challenge ourselves. Our bodies are wondrous in that they tell us when we're pushing to a new level: we become exhausted and we feel sore. There's a tension that's palpable when we're taking things farther than ever before.

Considering how far we've come in our quest to take control of our own health and fitness, the plateau of the "final 15" seems almost cruel. We've worked so hard—and still are working—not just in getting ourselves off the couch, but in changing what we eat and in making sure that we have the necessary support in our lives to achieve our goals.

When we do plateau, we look to our fitness, nutrition, and support coaches and ask, "Now what?" For countless weeks and months, we've eaten the same things and worked through the same routines, and every time we stepped on the scale the results were positive. But when those last pesky pounds won't fade away, though the days turn into weeks and the weeks turn into months, we become frustrated. We want to slack off—or, worse, quit. Because we've been attributing our overall success or failure to reaching a certain number (that old pesky focus on the destination), we feel like we'll never achieve the goals we originally set.

You *will* plateau if you don't recognize when you need to make a change. My advice: if a workout is routine and you can do it without breaking a sweat and without much thought, time to mix it up. Swim instead of run. Jump rope instead of use the StairMaster. Regardless of your exercise of choice, you have to be open to new, challenging workouts.

There's a key to breaking through a plateau, and the lesson can be learned from a characteristic of something found all around us—water. Water is a funny substance that changes its properties on a single degree of temperature. Keep water at 33 degrees, and it becomes very cold. Heat water to 211 degrees and it becomes very hot. But in either case, it remains essentially the same.

However, take water down one more degree—from 33 to 32 degrees—and it changes: it turns to ice. Take water up one degree—from 211 to 212—and it boils. When we reach a plateau in our own health and fitness, we're very good at getting to 33 or 211 degrees. We're very bad at taking it that one extra degree that makes the difference.

The health and fitness degree comes in many forms. Sometimes we need to change our workouts and challenge ourselves just that little bit more. Other times, we need to have the courage to increase the food we eat to ensure that our bodies have enough fuel to operate. Still other times, that one degree means we have to trust ourselves enough to know that while we're fallible human beings, the more our actual lifestyle changes, the less we have to find excuses to cheat when it comes to nutrition and fitness.

The key is to identify when that extra degree is necessary. For me, it was when I had lost 60 pounds, yet my progress had slowed for two weeks. I needed an extra degree. I needed to push myself beyond what I had been doing. Only then could I change.

I realized that I needed all of the elements mentioned above. I had to stop number crunching, mix up my workouts, and yes, eat more food. It took me a little while to realize what I needed, but once I did, I knew I would achieve my original goals. But more important than meeting my goals, I ended up with a perspective on weight loss and fitness that would improve my life in many ways beyond the physical.

When we plateau, our bodies are telling us that we're not doing enough to maintain our new lifestyle. It's like we're water at 211 degrees—pretty darn hot, but not quite boiling. We have to take the next leap of faith.

Only then will the true, systemic change that we desire (and that set us on our journey in the first place) be realized. Only then will we know what it means to find true health and fitness, this time for good.

Putting the "Life" in "Lifestyle"

There are a few things in life that can bond strangers together. When I was growing up, the most obvious one for me was sports. If you find a like-minded person who happens to share the same affinity for your team of choice, you become instant best friends, mocking the rest of the world for their poor choices.

Even if you meet someone who roots for your rival, you're suddenly bonded by the love of the game, and conversation flows about your given sport, the rivalry, and what's going to happen next.

Books can have the same effect. Lynn is an avid reader, and nothing seems to generate conversation like a shared novel. Indeed, groups of individuals organize book clubs for the opportunity to come together and speak about that shared interest (whether they agree or disagree on the quality of the writing).

There's a third fellowship that people join and immediately are welcomed into: parenthood. Nothing bonds people together like the chance to share war stories, provide advice, or seek guidance. Once you're a parent, you have an endless parade of fellow parents who can feel your pain and help you attempt to avoid the pitfalls they experienced.

While I used to think fondly of my daughters growing up and becoming independent, I now stare at the future of the teen years with angst and trepidation. My daughters have become ticking time bombs, inching closer to the inevitable tween and teen years.

As if I weren't already anxious enough about that upcoming transition, one fellow member of the parenthood club, Sarah, scared me to death. She is a parent, but it was a story of dealing with her parents that brought on a sobering reality.

Because we were all teenagers once, we know the tricks and arguments we used to torture our parents, so we try to protect our own children from themselves. Case in point, Sarah. She had two parents who approached her teenage years with an iron fist. Knowing what a teenager could pull, they tightened their grip on everything. They enforced significantly earlier curfews than other parents, made sure that their child came home every day to do homework, and made stalker-like efforts to find out what she was doing when the family was not together.

As is often the case with iron-fisted approaches, those efforts encouraged the opposite of what her parents had intended. The tighter they tried to manage her life, the more Sarah worked for her independence. To get around the curfew, she would sneak out the bedroom window. To keep her parents off the "scent," she had friends make up alibis. And as more restrictions were placed on her socializing, Sarah started choosing friends she knew would be exactly the opposite of her parents' wishes.

When I asked Sarah why things unfolded this way, she went right back to the iron fist. With that much control and restriction imposed on her, it felt natural to rebel and fight for her freedom. An adrenaline rush came with maneuvering around the restrictions and regulations. She felt justified breaking the rules.

Typical diet and fitness regimens thrive on similar restrictions. A specific diet can turn a piece of bread into "forbidden fruit," and fitness programs tend to spend as much time instructing participants on what *not* to do as they do on actual instruction for better health.

Early on, we follow along dutifully. After all, we made the choice to start. If we see results, it's easy to believe that the strict daily steps must be followed in perfect order or we won't keep getting results.

And for many, as we discussed, this seems to work—up until the point that results start to come at a slower (or nonexistent) pace. We're no longer seeing the pounds fall off or the inches disappear. Suddenly, we start seeing what we're missing—the lazy afternoons, the calorie-laden desserts, the forbidden fruit. Starting a program was our choice, but the tyranny of the program starts to lose its appeal. Freedom calls.

I want to pause here, because this is the point where most diet and fitness plans come to a screeching halt. That makes it worth another look. So . . . we begin with great intentions, energy, and drive. But at some point, we hit a plateau—a bump in the road. This critical moment leads to crashes of all sorts—from weekend binges to undoing everything we worked so hard for. So it's in this very moment that we must make a crucial choice. Is our diet about numbers and inches or is it about sustainable health? (Back to the destination vs. journey question again.) The wrong answer will lead us inevitably back to the beginning, and the right answer will guide us to the finish line—that is, living a healthy, fit life.

Here's how it unfolds.

When we're in the "militant" phase of a routine and the plateau takes hold, we become more perceptive regarding what we don't get to do or have. Suddenly, it feels as if every friend wants to enjoy an evening out at a calorie-exploding restaurant to celebrate every occasion.

Advertisements show up in the mail, offering two-for-one specials on the least special foods. And at the very moment that we're supposed to be heading to the gym, we find our favorite movie on television, begging us to curl up on the couch and take a break.

In spite of our best intentions, the rebellion against the diet or exercise plan subtly takes over. We rationalize that we've made such great progress that taking a weekend off isn't that bad. Monday comes along, and we decide that perhaps a full week off would help the body recover.

We sneak a cookie after dinner, as a reward for making it through another tough week, and have a cheat meal at a fast-food restaurant, though we're so guilt-ridden when we get home that we dispose of the fast-food trash in the bottom of our garbage can so nobody finds out.

Before we know it, we're in full rebellion, frustrated by a lack of results, addicted to the rush of forbidden treats, and tired of what we're clearly missing out on. The more our diet or fitness plan restricts us, the more we want to rebel when that plan isn't getting us closer to our goals. This is what I never understood pre-Fit2Fat2Fit.

When I was training James, his slipups were natural, normal, and expected. Instead of encouraging him through his choice and maybe offering strategies on how to handle the next temptation, I judged him and enforced stricter rules. Just like Sarah's parents, I was making it easier for James to rebel. Substitute my reaction to James with the restrictions of any diet or fitness plan and the results will be the same. Whether it was a meal plan telling James not to eat more than six ounces of protein for dinner, or a fitness routine listing the endless cardio elements necessary for the week, or a trainer unhappy that James had fallen off the wagon, the result was the same. James, like all of us, wanted freedom.

And that, inherently, is the problem. We follow plans that are so restrictive that they become the enemy, and we fight for our "freedom of choice" in what we're eating and how much we're working out. Taking on a new lifestyle, however, introduces a brand-new idea—that the key element of "lifestyle" is "life." As in, you actually have one, so live it.

Nutrition is, and will always be, about making the "right" choices every single day and at every meal. But there's no rulebook that says making the "wrong" choice every once in a while is going to kill your progress. In fact, it might actually help in the long run. The reality is that things come up—*life* comes up—and you'll be faced with difficult choices, decisions that might throw off your perfect diet or extensive workout routine.

I've always approached weekends with the acceptance that dietary splurges will likely occur and workout routines may be missed. And when they are missed, I move on. That's the key: moving on.

When we're on a diet or fitness plan that offers no flexibility or detours, every "wrong" choice feels like a loss. And the more we feel like failures, the less committed we are to trying to stay the course. When we take that diet or plan one step farther and actually change our lifestyle, we accept the fact that detours will happen, and a change for the better will come into effect at the very next meal or scheduled workout.

If I end up going out to a restaurant with friends and succumbing to a less-than-healthy dinner, I have a choice: to beat myself up about ordering a delicious hamburger and french fries, or to realize that it's now doubly important to eat the right meal the next morning. If an opportunity to spend the day with the family takes away a scheduled workout, I can feel guilty about skipping an important routine, or enjoy the family time, knowing that my schedule will allow the workout to happen the next day.

If a life is made up of making choices, the operative approach is to realize that "wrong" choices are a fact of life. Sustainable change occurs when we make many more "right" choices than "wrong" ones. When we give ourselves the freedom to roll with what life gives us, we also take away the adrenaline rush found in rebelling. We don't crave the need to give ourselves treats because we've been tortured without something for so long.

When we take that diet or plan one step farther and actually change our lifestyle, we accept the fact that detours will happen, and a change for the better will come into effect at the very next meal or scheduled workout.

And what happens next is one of life's miracles. Once we give ourselves freedom and flexibility, our choices start to become easier. Soon we find ourselves choosing the healthy option for dinner even when we go out—and realizing that it tastes great and makes us feel better than ever. Number crunching starts to disappear, and more and more right choices are made almost unconsciously. When we take away the restrictive diet plan or fitness routine, our choices become less about weight or pants size and more about looking and feeling great—that is, about a healthy lifestyle.

As I finished talking with my fellow parent, Sarah, the one whose parents had been so strict, I asked her how she was going to be a different parent when her kids got to the teenage years. Her answer was simple. "I'll let them act like teenagers."

In the fight to be healthy, maybe it's time we let ourselves act like human beings.

CONCLUSION

IT'S A LIFESTYLE, NOT A DIET

The alarm on my phone wakes me up, the first step of my new daily routine. I roll over and see that my wife is still deeply asleep. It looks as if she hasn't moved all night, and I doubt she will for the next hour as I start my day. I glance over at the clock, realizing that I have another 30 minutes before the house is filled with waking children.

I quickly brush my teeth, shower, shave, and begin the surprisingly difficult process of finding something to wear. I dig through my old clothes, first trying pants. The ones I've been used to over the last year are all now dangerously close to falling to my ankles, but I find a workable pair and belt them firmly on. I sit on the corner of the bed and quickly tie my shoes, the days of being out of breath long gone.

I move to the mirror to check my ensemble. If I hadn't lived it myself, I would never know I'd gained and lost 75 pounds over the last year. My reflection in the mirror is the same as when I started this personal journey, and yet I'm so clearly different.

When I've had personal struggles—events in the past that have shaken me to the core—I've internalized them. Unconsciously, I've tried to hide the turmoil and the resulting changes from others.

I lived through the loss of a job, for example, and still clearly remember the feelings of inadequacy. That experience has happened to many people, of course, and I discovered, when I joined the club of those who've lost their ability to provide for their families, that I'm forever bonded to those who have lived through it as well.

A friend of mine, in what clearly must have been a moment of weakness (we guys don't talk about this stuff), related to me his own experience at being let go from a job. He talked about the difficulty of portraying a calm public face while everything that he knew crumbled around him.

Mike's loss of a job hadn't been expected. He was happily employed and seemed to be thriving at work. One Monday morning he was told, out of the blue, that his services were no longer required. As Mike started the drive home, fear engulfed him. How would he make sure that his child had enough to eat? What would he say to break the news to his unassuming wife?

Mike allowed himself one breakdown; he wept as he told his life partner what had happened. Then he stiffened his resolve to find a better job. He would turn this into an opportunity, he decided. He applied for jobs in droves, convinced that he would rebound immediately.

That was Mike's outward face. As time dragged on and no opportunities presented themselves, his inward view started to shift. He found himself lying on his bedroom floor, staring into oblivion as hours passed by. It took every last bit of strength and perseverance within him to keep applying for jobs, as every rejection made the experience more hopeless.

Yet as the search for employment became more unbearable, Mike found light and meaning elsewhere. His extra time at home created a greater bond with his child. He started helping around the house. He couldn't believe the level of unwavering support his wife provided.

These happy moments were subtle, but potent. Mike soon found himself more focused in the job hunt and interview process. He had found a new base of strength and support, and that changed the way he viewed potential work situations.

After long months, an opportunity did present itself. The new position was a better fit for the man he was becoming, as Mike started to let go of his guilt at "failing" his family in the first place. Before long, he found himself back in the routine of a new job, seeing his family only in the evenings.

And yet something had changed. The checks were again coming in, but Mike wasn't the same person. The experience had changed him for the better, even if it seemed at the time that nothing good could have come from it.

Months after I'd decided to gain weight for the experience of losing it again, I found myself in a strange state of hopelessness. I wondered what I had done to my family, my life, and myself. Privately, I questioned whether I would really be able to make my way back.

At first what plagued me most was the fear of not truly knowing what I was getting into and how I was going to make it to the other side. Then the shock followed—the shock to my confidence and sense of self as the experience changed my relationship to the outside world.

But beyond the fear on one side and the confidence on the other, a bigger shift was taking place. I no longer saw the world in black and white. Finally, I understood that I had been wrong about why we make the choices we do (or don't) as related to our health. That understanding enriched me both as a person and as a personal trainer.

This change in perception would never have happened had I not realized and acknowledged who I was in the three stages of this experience—fit, then fat, then fit again—and how every stage impacted the man who rolled out of bed in the mornings.

From Fit . . .

Before the journey, I saw health as a physical state of being, one that could be reached and maintained with what I then described in simplified motivational sound bites like "determination," "choice," and "devotion."

If you'd asked my wife or close friends to describe my approach in those days, they'd have mentioned physical products—weights, spinach, treadmills.

Months before my journey began, Lynn and I had gone to dinner at a friend's house. After a delicious meal with wonderful conversation, we all settled down to watch movies and relax. While the others in the group started to salivate over typical late-night movie snacks, I sat in the corner and gave my attention to the TV screen. The smell of popcorn couldn't tempt me.

My friend, however, had another idea. Carrots. She brought me a whole bowl of them. If nothing else, it was a thoughtful gesture which illustrated that my friends and family understood my devotion to proper nutrition.

Back then, however, I was overly focused on avoiding foods that were "high-carb." I tended to avoid root vegetables such as carrots because of their high starch content.

So instead of taking the carrots and appreciating the gesture, I answered with a matter-of-fact, "Thanks, but carrots are too high-carb for me." My friend couldn't decide if I was being humorous or just plain rude.

She walked away deflated. My friends and my wife proceeded to mock me for the rest of the evening. Back then, with every joke at my expense, I felt more justified in my stance—more self-righteous, if you will. Now, I can laugh at myself.

In my personal training work, I tried to impart the wisdom that I felt so strongly about to the people who were overweight. Instead of easing them into small changes, I walked them through a whole encyclopedia of good and bad fruits, rich and poor vegetables. In my own mind, this approach to fitness seemed reasonable. And I pushed exercise. I wasn't going to make one of my clients keel over, of course, so we'd start with the basics, like push-ups and planks. I was sure that sore muscles would directly result in stronger commitment.

Everything I stood for and all my actions were based on the belief that people were in their current state (whether fit or not) because they chose to be so. If someone was struggling with his or her own health and fitness, that person simply needed to choose change. My meal plans and fitness routines would do the rest.

My successes in personal training—and there were some significant ones—galvanized my militant approach. Any failures were excused due to my clients' lack of conviction. They obviously weren't trying hard enough.

I simply couldn't understand why people made decisions that negatively affected their health. Healthy living requires healthy choices. My reaction to a friendly bowl of carrot sticks was more telling of who I was as a person than of the kind of trainer I tried to be (even if I didn't really see it at the time). I was so blinded by my own views on health that I couldn't understand anything on the "other side" of the argument. And that's exactly what needed to change; the bodily changes were secondary. Because I was healthy, fit, militant . . . but woefully ignorant.

To Fat . . .

It happened just weeks before the fit portion of the journey was to begin. Lynn had waited until the kids were asleep and we were sitting alone at the dining room table. It was unlike her to corner me when I was least expecting it. But I sensed that something was coming—a message I was afraid to hear.

My thoughts leading up to the confrontation kept taking me back to a moment of clarity at the grocery store months before. My visits each week had become routine. I had expertly charted a course through the aisles that took me past my favorite foods. I spent extra time in the soda aisle, which was conveniently placed near my weekly ration of Zingers. A few paces away, I'd find my Cinnamon Toast Crunch. I was well beyond the days of forcing myself to enjoy processed foods; I had already begun to fear the time when they wouldn't be allowed in my grocery cart.

As I started unloading my cart at the checkout line, three women stood behind me. Was I imagining their stares as I pulled all my "necessities" out of the cart? I was sure I could feel their eyes moving from my bulging waistline to the conveyor belt. I could sense their silent judgment, thoughts like *No wonder he's fat* and *How many liters of Mountain Dew does one person need?*

I had already started hating any trips out of the house, because I felt self-conscious about everything from my gait to the size of my hips and buttocks. I felt like less of a person the bigger I got, as if I'd lost a bit of what made me . . . well, *me*. As I walked away from the store that day, I realized that being overweight wasn't all about the waistline. It was about self-worth, and the reality that the world looked down on you without even knowing your story. That was a lot harder to deal with than a couple of bench presses had ever been.

Less than a month later, another realization hit. This one was closer to home. While I don't think I ever underestimated the energy level of my two-year-old daughter, Kale'a, I'm quite sure that it had increased at the same rate that my energy level had plummeted.

It was such a simple game for her: she would run through the house and Daddy would try to catch her. Yet a few laps in that day, the chafing started. The tightening of my lungs and loss of breath took whatever fight I had left. I sat down exhausted and told my daughter that the three minutes of playtime were all she was going to get. She looked directly into my eyes as tears filled hers. As the tears spilled over, she searched for her mother for consolation. She'd have to find a better playmate.

How had a dietary experiment led to me disappointing my daughter? This was not the father I wanted to be. My previous assumptions had been totally shattered. There was a sense of entrapment in the added weight, now pulling down both my body and my attitude. It seemed that a decision to eat what I wanted and avoid exercise in favor of a more sedentary lifestyle had resulted in bad choices now being stronger than I was. And the effects went beyond me: there were other casualties in the war I had waged on my health.

This brings me back to my conversation with Lynn, who spoke so calmly it was unnerving. She talked about the journey from her perspective, and about the effects I'd been too blind to see. After over six years of marriage and two children, it was unbearable to hear my spouse say she didn't recognize me anymore. It was even more unsettling when I realized it had nothing to do with my physical appearance.

Lynn talked about the added burden of keeping up with the house, the chores, and errands as my contributions fell off. She explained that she felt like a single parent, faced with a newborn and a two-year-old.

I knew Lynn said what she did only because she loved me. She had to be honest so that her feelings wouldn't turn into resentment. But I couldn't say anything in return. There was no defense; there was no justification.

I was fat, but I was no longer shallow. At least not shallow enough to think that weight was an exclusively physical malady. In fact, the weight itself could be managed to some extent. There were powders for chafing, lotions for stretch marks, antacids for the ailing stomach, and nose strips for the snoring.

But there was no lotion that could combat the depression that had crept into my life. I couldn't buy a powder to appease the disappointment of my child at my physical limitations. And antacids wouldn't take away the feeling that my wife had come to regard me as a stranger in her house.

I couldn't buy a powder to appease the disappointment of my child at my physical limitations. And antacids wouldn't take away the feeling that my wife had come to regard me as a stranger in her house.

Being overweight wasn't a lazy person's decision not to try. It was a symptom of a struggle within a person's emotional and mental life that transcended the physical being. Simultaneously, it was a war with society as a whole.

I was just scratching the surface of the many factors that made getting and staying healthy difficult. Everyone's battles are different, but I was beginning to finally understand the scope of the problem.

With this deeper understanding, I turned my thoughts to my pending transition from Fat-2Fit. Would I be caught in the same pattern? My journey was always meant to be temporary, but I was afraid I was stuck.

To Fit

There's an old saying that doctors make the worst patients. Having worked in that industry, I've heard my fair share of stories proving that true. On one hand, you'd think that the knowledge and experience a doctor can provide would make him or her a good partner in treatment. The patient-doctor could consult and discuss, and the adage that "two heads are better than one" would certainly prove true.

Yet that's the opposite of what seems to happen. When a doctor becomes the patient, the result is generally a battle of wills. There's a competition for who is right and who is wrong, and if there are various solutions to the problem, the actual doctor will have to prove why his or her treatment protocol is the right one.

I can attest that this adage crosses over into the gym. There's nothing like trying to take instruction from another personal trainer. If a fellow gym rat attempts to correct your form, you tend to do it your way with even more vigor. When presented with workout routines and meal plans from other personal trainers, you spend your time picking their choices apart because they clearly don't understand what true health is.

My decision to forgo exercise for the first month of my Fat2Fit journey was a calculated one. I knew that the key to any weight-loss program was nutrition, so I dove into my calculated plan without worrying about push-ups or pull-ups initially.

And while it took multiple months of gaining weight to start having my "aha" moments, it took only a single day on the weight-loss side to realize I had miscalculated already. Because the moment I removed Mountain Dew from my daily intake, my body revolted.

I used to scoff at clients who complained about missing their sodas (even the diet versions were forbidden) and about the severe withdrawal headaches that would ensue. I thought it was just an excuse to fall off the wagon. And yet here I was, groaning on the couch when my soda headaches commenced. The throbbing was persistent and painful, and I lost any motivation to move from my sedentary state. I resisted the urge to fuel my addiction, but the sheer fact that I considered it was alarming and frightening.

I finally understood what my clients kept telling me: stepping away from a lifetime of bad nutrition and poor choices was not just a question of making that first decision.

My mind was working against me. And yet I persevered. As time passed, my body got reacquainted with my spinach shake and other recipes. The headaches faded away, but the lessons remained. I finally understood what my clients kept telling me: stepping away from a lifetime of bad nutrition and poor choices was *not* just a question of making that first decision.

Every such lesson came with a sense of humility not often seen in the personal training profession. I was horrified to learn how wrong I'd been, even as I tried to be helpful.

As a personal trainer, I could always see that some of my clients weren't capable of pushing themselves adequately. If they were, why would they need a trainer in the first place? I had to take them to the next level for their own good, not just during our sessions but during our follow-up calls and conversations.

When I sat down to design my own Fat2Fit program, I was ambitious. I knew what my fitness levels had been just seven months previously, and this was my chance to prove that, when motivated, I could accomplish great things. Especially because I knew about muscle memory. Yet by the time I got to the gym, I wasn't an ambitious personal trainer. I wasn't even an enthusiastic client.

The self-doubt that had crept into my mind as my body changed was still omnipresent. Even worse, when I did walk through the gym doors and saw my picture on a bulletin board (an old Fit2Fat2Fit journey flyer), I could feel my ego shrinking. I wanted to disappear into a back corner; I didn't want anyone to check my form or see my struggles.

For the first time in my life, I was doing push-ups on my knees—and barely surviving the process. Halfway through my workout, my legs felt as though they were going to give out. My psyche wasn't doing much better.

I was caught between how much I'd lost in the last seven months and how hard the trek back was going to be. And I saw the world through my clients' eyes, thinking there wasn't any reason for encouragement in barely finishing a set of exercises. And don't get me started on the shame in having to drop to my knees just to get through. Working out wasn't a display of possibilities now; it was a reminder of just how unmanageable every little step felt. If the first six months of my journey had shown me how my weight gain could put an emotional strain on my wife, children, and other loved ones, I wasn't prepared for the level of support I would need in crawling back.

On a daily basis, I had to struggle to get motivated. My wife would literally push me off the couch to get me to the gym. I'd have moments when I wanted to cheat on my nutritional plan. My wife would be making a cake, and I'd let various strategies roll through my head as to how I could steal a piece. Surely I could restart my trip back to health the *next* day.

I was caught between how much I'd lost in the last seven months and how hard the trek back was going to be. I saw the world through my clients' eyes, thinking there wasn't any reason for encouragement in barely finishing a set of exercises.

Yet behind every moment of weakness, there was an e-mail—a story from a follower who told me to keep going and take it one day at a time. These messages reminded me about how we motivate each other, strengthening our resolve to take charge of our own health.

And that, in the end, was the biggest lesson of all. This wasn't just about eating the right foods or following the proper workout plan anymore. I ultimately understood what people meant when they spoke about finding balance—a healthy balance between nutrition, fitness, persistence, and support. It was about finding creative ways to push yourself physically and mentally and searching out new resources. It was the realization that the journey from Fat2Fit is one you take with others. You need to surround yourself with people who will ensure that you keep getting with the program.

I'm usually greeted with two waves of responses to Fit2Fat2Fit. Initially people barrage me with superficial inquiries ranging from the size of my hips to the craziest food challenge I attempted. In a way, everyone is interested in what it would be like to live with an unrestricted diet and avoidance of physical activity.

Only after going through the whole cycle of last year did I realize that their inquiries almost always started where my own journey began—in the physical. Perhaps that's because it's painfully obvious: there's no getting around the rotund belly I had developed. But maybe it's also because, deep down, anyone who has been overweight knows that the real battle lies in the emotional and mental difficulties presented.

When the first wave of inquiries fades, questions change in tone. People begin to ask how I felt about myself as a heavy person, how my family fared, and other such internal matters. In other words, they get down to those emotional and mental difficulties.

As I made my way from Fit2Fat2Fit, daily stories from my Twitter feed and Facebook postings told other people's stories. I was inspired by a man who readily admitted to falling off the nutritional wagon during a vacation, only to come back more committed and drop seven pounds in a single week. I found hope in the stories of followers who were able to keep up with their children, mow their own lawn, or start teaching their family how to eat and be healthy.

I learned that in order to overcome my own weight gain, I had to first accept that the journey would challenge me physically, mentally, and emotionally. I couldn't stick to my old patterns on my way back. There was a level of mental and physical balance required to reach my goals and value my goals at the same time.

The ultimate question: Was it worth it?

It could be argued that nothing was gained or lost in my journey, from a physical standpoint. I started with a 34-inch waist and ended with the same. My reflection was eerily similar (even manscaping had resumed!) after the final transformation to what it had been 365 days prior.

But emotionally and mentally, I'm living a different life. It's amazing what you take for granted when you're healthy (and have been for as long as you can remember). Even the simple joys of housework become a big deal when taken away.

My oldest daughter now seems to be in a perpetual good mood because I can't get enough of chasing her. I look forward to being able to do the same with my one-year-old.

Every date with my wife holds extra meaning, as I realize what gaining 75 pounds nearly took away from me, and what losing 75 pounds gave me back. (Answer: my life.) And that's what makes every step worth it. I now realize that my health has a direct effect on those around me, and I'll never forget that they stuck with me and encouraged me to complete my journey. With each new client, I will emphasize the focus on community. I cannot repeat its importance enough.

Beyond my wife and family, however, lies a group of individuals who made every meal plan, workout routine, withdrawal from Mountain Dew, and tough-love session from my wife worth it beyond anything I could have imagined. It's the people who joined me on the journey from Fat2Fit2Fat.

I now believe that every e-mail, letter, and vote on a web poll played a crucial role. Those who challenged me strengthened my resolve to complete the cycle and be open to the lessons that could come, even when I didn't want to learn them. Those who showed the courage to take on my meal plans and workout routines themselves kept me accountable. I couldn't slack off or cheat: they would know—and so would I. The Fit2Fat2Fit community made me realize that you never go it alone when it comes to health and fitness, but instead fight through together.

A grand total of 365 days. Six months of unrestricted diet and absolutely no working out, followed by six more months of food withdrawal, prepared meals, cruel workouts, and a never-ending support network.

A single journey from Fit2Fat2Fit. But perhaps more accurately, a journey from Fit2Fat2 . . . *changed*—in every possible way.

My yearlong odyssey was an extreme, of course. Gaining weight intentionally and then trying to lose it in a tight schedule was what I felt I needed to do to understand the struggles so many of us face with our health. Throughout this process, my very specific journey led to some universal takeaways.

Some of us might need to lose 15 pounds. Some may be looking just to get into better physical shape. Some have been struggling with weight all their lives. It doesn't matter where you are when you start. It matters *that* you start. Everyone is on their own journey.

During the many days when I struggled, I always hoped I would come to the end of this journey with something of value to pass on. I started this odyssey to equip myself to better help others and soon learned that I was the one who needed help. I could never have done this alone.

Perhaps the biggest lesson, and the one I want to leave with you here at the end, is to *share your experience*. It may be with a family member, a key friend, a strong community, a trainer (one who understands!), or online. It doesn't matter who—it just matters that you don't attempt the journey by yourself. You can accomplish all your health goals and change your life for good, as long as you've got support behind you and the courage to declare your own journey.

If you share your goals and are honest about your challenges, you will find that you have all the resources and support needed to succeed. I know you can. The time is now; the decision is yours.

RECIPES

Pumpkin Pie Protein Shake

Makes 1 serving

1 scoop Protein2Fit Vanilla Whey Protein Isolate

½ cup unsweetened almond milk

1 banana

¼ cup canned pumpkin puree

⅛ teaspoon nutmeg

¼ teaspoon cinnamon

¼ teaspoon vanilla

1 packet sugar substitute (such as Stevia or Splenda)

3 handfuls ice

Blend ingredients together and enjoy!

The Best Spinach Shake Ever

Makes 1 serving

1 scoop Protein2Fit Vanilla Whey Protein Isolate

3 cups fresh spinach

½ banana

2 tablespoons peanut butter (preferably natural)

¾ cup unsweetened almond milk

2 cups ice

Combine these items in a blender, and you're ready to go! This delicious, quick, healthy drink (featured on *The Dr. Oz Show*) is packed with quality protein, good fat, plenty of potassium, a dose of vitamin C, and beneficial fiber. This shake can be used as a great breakfast, lunch, dinner, or pre/postworkout meal; alternatively, you can halve the recipe and enjoy the shake as one of your snacks during the day. To make this extra-low in carbs, omit the banana.

Spinach Egg-White Omelet

Makes 1 serving

½ cup egg whites (from about 3 large eggs) and 1 whole egg

¼ cup chopped onions

2 tablespoons chopped jalapeños (optional)

½ cup fresh spinach

¼ cup chopped mushrooms

¼ cup chopped red bell pepper

½ cup precooked chicken breast

2 tablespoons salsa

Spray a medium-size skillet with olive oil nonstick spray. Mix the egg whites and whole egg together. Once the pan reaches medium-high heat, add the eggs and wait 30 seconds. Then add the onions, jalapeños, spinach, mushrooms, red bell pepper, and chicken breast, placing them in a line along the middle. Once the eggs start to bubble and become firm on the bottom (usually 1 to 2 minutes), indicating that the omelet is ready to flip, sprinkle the outside edges with water using your fingertips—as it bubbles it creates a space that helps make it easier to use a spatula for flipping. Flip/close the omelet and cook for another minute or so; then flip the omelet to the other side for another 1 to 2 minutes, or until done. Once the omelet is cooked to your liking, serve with the salsa on top and enjoy.

Egg-White Breakfast Burrito

Makes 1 serving   Prep: 10 minutes   Cook: 5 minutes

- ½ cup egg whites (from about 3 large eggs) and 1 whole egg
- ¼ cup chopped cauliflower
- ¼ cup chopped yellow bell pepper
- ¼ cup chopped mushrooms
- ½ cup fresh spinach
- ½ cup precooked chicken breast
- 1 low-carb tortilla
- 2 tablespoons salsa
- ¼ cup chopped avocado (optional)

Spray a medium-size skillet with olive oil nonstick spray. Mix the egg whites and whole egg together. Add the egg mixture to the preheated pan on medium-high heat and stir continuously until the eggs are thoroughly cooked (usually 3 to 4 minutes). Then add the vegetables and chicken. Top with salsa and avocado and wrap in a low-carb tortilla. Anything that doesn't fit in the tortilla, eat by itself.

Farmer's Breakfast Scramble

Makes 1 serving   Prep: 10 minutes   Cook: 5 minutes

½ cup egg whites (from about 3 large eggs) and 1 whole egg
½ cup precooked brown rice
¼ cup chopped onions
¼ cup chopped red bell pepper
¼ cup chopped mushrooms
½ cup fresh spinach
2 slices turkey lunch meat

Spray a medium-size skillet with olive oil nonstick spray. Mix the egg whites and whole egg together. Add the egg mixture to the preheated pan on medium-high heat and stir continuously until the eggs are thoroughly cooked (usually 3 to 4 minutes). Then add the brown rice, vegetables, and turkey meat. Other lunch meat can be substituted for the turkey, if you prefer.

Chinese "Fried Rice"

Makes 4 to 6 servings   Prep: 10 minutes   Cook: 15 minutes

10 ounces fresh cauliflower (about ½ medium head)
Cooking oil
3 green onions, sliced and roughly separated into green and white
1 clove garlic, minced
Dash of ginger, optional
3 tablespoons soy sauce
Few drops of sesame oil, to taste
2 cups raw shrimp, peeled
3 eggs, beaten

Grate the cauliflower using either the largest holes on a hand grater or the grating blade in a food processor. The results should resemble cooked white rice—hence the recipe's name. Weigh out 10 ounces of the grated cauliflower and reserve remaining florets (I had four good-size pieces left) for another use. On medium-high, heat enough oil to cover the bottom of a wok or large skillet. Quickly stir-fry the garlic and the white of the onions. Watch closely so as not to burn. Add the cauliflower; fry about 4 to 5 minutes, stirring constantly, until it begins to color a bit. Don't overcook or it will get mushy. Stir in the ginger, soy sauce, sesame oil, onion greens, and shrimp. Stir-fry until shrimp turn pink and are cooked through. Push the "rice" mixture to one side of the wok. Pour the eggs into the other side; scramble and cook until still moist. Mix the eggs into the "rice," breaking up any large chunks of egg.

Tip: This dish stores and reheats well.

Sun-Dried Tomato Chicken

Makes 4 servings Prep: 10 minutes Cook: 10 minutes

4 boneless, skinless chicken breasts
8 tablespoons Tuscan Sun-Dried Tomato Marinade

Cut chicken into small cubes. Spray a large skillet with nonstick cooking spray. Heat skillet to medium-high. Add chicken to the skillet and immediately add all the marinade on top of the chicken and stir in. The marinade will cook into the chicken to add more flavor. Cook chicken, stirring occasionally until it is completely cooked through (not pink in the middle of the chicken).

Tip: For better flavor, marinate chicken overnight. If you can't find sun-dried tomato marinade at your grocery store, feel free to substitute a different marinade that's low in sugar.

BBQ Chicken Lettuce Wraps

Makes 8 servings   Prep: 20 minutes   Cook: 60 minutes

3 pounds boneless, skinless chicken breasts
BBQ sauce of your choosing (preferably one low in sugar)
1 large head iceberg lettuce
1 red onion, chopped (optional)
1 or 2 large carrots, grated (optional)

Preheat oven to 400°F. Line a 9 × 13-inch glass baking dish with aluminum foil. Spray foil with olive oil (or other) nonstick spray. Place chicken in baking dish (as many pieces as you can fit in, because leftovers will be useful over the next few days). Spoon your favorite BBQ sauce over the chicken until all the pieces are covered. Bake for 50 to 60 minutes, until chicken is no longer pink inside. Carefully shred the cooked meat into whole leaves of the iceberg lettuce, using the leaves as "wraps" to place the chicken in. Tuck shredded carrots and red onion in with the chicken, if you'd like, and enjoy.

Tip: This meal is even tastier if the chicken is prepared in a slow cooker. The meat is more tender that way, and the sauce has more time to simmer into the chicken.

Roast Chicken

Makes 4 servings   Prep: 10 minutes   Cook: 20–25 minutes

½ teaspoon sea salt (optional)
¾ teaspoon fennel seeds, crushed
¼ teaspoon freshly ground black pepper
¼ teaspoon garlic powder
¼ teaspoon dried oregano
4 boneless, skinless chicken breasts (4 to 6 ounces each)
6 teaspoons olive oil, divided
1 large shallot, thinly sliced
2 teaspoons chopped fresh rosemary
2 medium red bell peppers, thinly sliced
1 yellow bell pepper, thinly sliced
1 cup chicken broth
1 tablespoon balsamic vinegar

Preheat oven to 450°F. Combine salt, crushed fennel seeds, freshly ground black pepper, garlic powder, and oregano. Brush chicken with 2 teaspoons olive oil and sprinkle the spice rub over the meat. Heat a large skillet over medium-high heat and add 2 teaspoons olive oil. Add chicken and cook 3 minutes, or until browned. Turn each piece and cook 1 minute more. Remove chicken from the skillet and arrange pieces in a large baking dish. Bake for 15 to 20 minutes, or until fully cooked.

Meanwhile, heat remaining olive oil over medium-high heat in the same large skillet used to brown the chicken (without washing the pan first). When the pan is hot, add shallots and rosemary and sauté 3 to 5 minutes, or until shallot pieces are translucent. Add peppers and stir in broth, scraping the pan to loosen brown bits. Reduce heat and simmer 5 minutes. Add vinegar and season with additional sea salt and freshly ground black pepper. Cook 3 minutes more, stirring frequently. Serve sauce over chicken.

Mexican Chicken

Makes 4 servings   Prep: 20 minutes   Cook: 50–60 minutes

1 pound boneless, skinless chicken breasts
1 teaspoon prepared taco seasoning
½ cup red enchilada sauce
1 small can chopped black olives
1 small can chopped green chilies
4 ounces cheddar cheese, shredded (optional)
3 green onions, chopped

Sprinkle the chicken on both sides with taco seasoning; grill or sauté. Cut the cooked chicken into cubes and place in a greased 8 × 8-inch baking dish. Add the enchilada sauce and toss the chicken to coat. Sprinkle the cheese (optional) and olives over the chicken and bake at 350°F for 10 to 20 minutes, until hot and bubbly. Scatter the green chilies and green onions over the top.

Basil Chicken with Vegetables

Makes 2 to 3 servings   Prep: 10 minutes   Cook: 10 minutes

1 pound boneless, skinless chicken breasts, cut into bite-size pieces
1 red bell pepper, chopped
8 ounces mushrooms, sliced
2 cups sliced zucchini or other summer squash
8 ounces fresh basil, chopped
3 cloves garlic, minced or pressed
3 tablespoons olive oil
Salt and pepper to taste

Heat oil in a large skillet on high heat. Sprinkle salt and pepper on the chicken before placing it in the skillet. Cook chicken on one side and then turn the pieces over. Add the vegetables and stir. When food is nearly cooked, push it to one side and add the garlic. After about 30 seconds, stir all those ingredients together and add the basil. Cook another 30 to 60 seconds and serve.

Tip: Pesto (homemade or store-bought) can be substituted for the garlic and basil.

Cajun Chicken Stir-Fry

Makes 2 to 4 servings   *Prep: 5 minutes*   *Cook: 10 minutes*

2 boneless, skinless chicken breasts, cut into strips
1 teaspoon spicy seasoning salt
1 large red bell pepper, cut into strips
1 small onion, slivered
1 clove garlic, minced
Oil and/or butter
Salt and pepper to taste

In a small bowl, toss the raw chicken with the seasoning to coat. Heat a small amount of oil and/or butter in a large skillet on medium-high. Sauté the chicken, red pepper, onion, and garlic until the chicken is cooked through and the pepper pieces are crisp-tender. Season with additional salt and pepper to taste.

Thai Turkey Skillet

Makes 4 servings   Prep: 15 minutes   Cook: 15 minutes

1 pound lean ground turkey
2 red bell peppers, thinly sliced
2 tablespoons minced or grated fresh ginger
3 cloves garlic, chopped
1 teaspoon red pepper flakes
3 tablespoons peanut butter (preferably natural)
2 tablespoons lime juice
2 tablespoons soy sauce
1 tablespoon sesame oil
½ cup cilantro, chopped
8 romaine lettuce leaves

Brown the ground turkey in a large nonstick skillet or wok; drain the grease. Add the peppers, ginger, garlic, and red pepper flakes. Cook over medium-high heat about 4 minutes, or until the peppers have softened slightly. Meanwhile, whisk together the peanut butter, lime juice, soy sauce, sesame oil, and cilantro. Remove the skillet from the heat and add the peanut butter mixture to the skillet; mix well. Serve the meat mixture rolled up in the lettuce leaves (or, if you prefer, over chopped lettuce).

Turkey Breast and Berry Salad

Makes 1 serving

4 slices turkey lunch meat, cut up
1 handful almonds
1 handful blueberries
1 handful strawberries
3 cups mixed dark salad greens
2 tablespoons purchased or homemade light raspberry vinaigrette dressing

Arrange the lettuce and berries on a plate, add the turkey pieces, and top with salad dressing.

Tip: This can be made with any type of lunch meat you prefer.

Beef Fajitas

Makes 4 servings *Prep: 5 minutes* *Cook: 10 minutes*

1½ pounds frozen, seasoned beef fajita meat (or you can substitute fresh beef flank steak or carne asada with 1 package of fajita seasoning)
1 cup red bell pepper
1 cup white onion
½ cup salsa
½ of an avocado

Cook fajita meat in a medium to large skillet. Once the meat is defrosted and almost fully cooked, add in the peppers and onions for an additional two minutes. Remove from the heat and add in the salsa and avocado. Stir together and enjoy.

Caramelized Onion–Glazed Salmon

Makes 4 servings *Prep: 5 minutes* *Cook: 30 minutes*

4 salmon fillets (about 6 ounces each)
1 white onion, thinly sliced
8 slices precooked turkey bacon, cut into thirds
⅓ cup low-calorie brown sugar

Preheat oven to 350°F. Spray a 9 × 13-inch baking pan with cooking spray. Place salmon fillets in the bottom, topped by slices of onion. Next, layer each salmon piece with turkey bacon and sprinkle with low-calorie brown sugar. Cover the top of the pan with foil and cook for 20 minutes. Remove foil and bake for 10 more minutes, or until salmon is cooked all the way through.

Citrus Salmon with Avocado Salsa

Makes 4 servings *Prep: 45 minutes* *Cook: 6–8 minutes*

4 salmon fillets (about 6 ounces each)
½ tablespoon olive oil
4 tablespoons fresh orange juice
1 teaspoon sea salt
1 teaspoon onion powder
1 teaspoon paprika
½ teaspoon black pepper
⅓ teaspoon allspice
⅓ teaspoon cayenne pepper

Avocado Salsa

1 large avocado, diced
½ cup diced red onion
1 orange, peeled, sectioned, and diced
1 jalapeño pepper, seeded, ribs removed, and diced, *or* ⅓ teaspoon cayenne pepper

2 teaspoons fresh lime juice
3 tablespoons fresh orange juice
2 tablespoons fresh cilantro, minced
Sea salt and black pepper to taste

In a baking dish, combine the olive oil and the orange juice. Lay salmon in it and turn to coat. In a small bowl, combine the salt, onion powder, paprika, black pepper, allspice, and cayenne pepper. Sprinkle those spices over each side of the salmon fillets. Set fish aside to marinate for 30 minutes.

Meanwhile, in a small bowl, combine all ingredients listed above for Avocado Salsa. Mix, cover, and chill in the refrigerator until ready to use.

Lightly coat a large skillet with olive oil (or other) nonstick spray and heat the pan to medium-high. Add the salmon and cook for 4 to 5 minutes; turn fillets and cook on the other side for 2 to 3 minutes, or until fish flakes easily. Serve with chilled Avocado Salsa.

Sea Salt Salmon with Olive Oil Mayo

Makes 4 servings   Prep: 5 minutes   Cook: 30 minutes

4 salmon fillets (about 6 ounces each)
8 tablespoons purchased olive oil mayo
Dash of sea salt

Preheat oven to 350°F. Place salmon fillets on individual pieces of foil (sized to allow wrapping of each). Spread each salmon piece with 2 tablespoons olive oil mayo and sprinkle with sea salt before tightly closing the foil around each. Put the foil packets in a 9 × 13-inch pan. Place the pan in the oven and bake the fillets for 20 minutes. Open the foil packets and bake 10 more minutes, or until salmon is cooked.

MEAL PLANS

Meal Plan 1: The Beginning

The following monthlong meal plan is designed to jump-start your weight loss and change your unhealthy eating habits. For me, it was easier to make these changes while doing no formal workouts—only stretching and core exercises. I didn't go to the gym at all during this phase, but instead focused on breaking some bad eating habits and cleansing my body of toxins from processed foods.

This meal plan cuts out dairy and grains in order to cut out the majority of fats and carbohydrates and help prevent digestive problems. The meal plan instead focuses on lean meats, fresh veggies, and fruits. In essence, I used a similar version of this for the first month on my journey from Fat2Fit. This may be a drastic change in most people's eating regimen, but everyone I know of who has committed to following this for 30 days has seen not only weight loss but an increase in energy, as well as medical health benefits (improved levels of blood pressure, cholesterol, glucose, and testosterone).

As I mentioned earlier, I believe that we should eat approximately every three hours throughout the day, rather than simply three times daily. The purposes of eating every three hours is to keep your metabolism running, blood sugar levels steady, and to keep you satisfied throughout the day, to help prevent binge eating. Obviously, schedules for all of us are different, but the goal is to achieve a balanced regimen. My meal plans account for that more frequent intake of food.

For all the entrées listed in the meal plans, a recipe is provided in the appendix titled "Recipes," preceding this one. You can substitute one recipe for another on any day, as long as the new recipe contributes about the same number of calories and nutrients.

I created these meal plans for myself; thus they reflect a male's caloric needs. If you're a woman, I would recommend that you make a slight adjustment in the number of calories consumed per day on each plan. You can mix and match as you see fit, but in general reduce the overall daily caloric intake by about 400 calories. This can be done with portion size or by cutting out one of the snacks (or via a combination of anything that works well for you). Remember: the goal is balance.

Note that with entrées, the caloric count is given before any side dish is named. Calories from veggies are relatively low (less than 75 calories on average for 2 cups of steamed veggies), so we included them in the total calories.

You may notice that there are no built-in cheat/treat meals this month, as there are in the next meal plan. This is to help break through food addictions.

Finally, you will see a number of supplements listed below. My brands of choice are the following: Protein2Fit Whey Protein Isolate, Multi2Fit Whole Food Vitamin, and Enzymes2Fit Daily Digestive Enzymes (digestive enzymes "unlock" the nutritional value in our foods; aid in breaking down our food into their smallest components for optimal absorption of vitamins, minerals, and other nutrients; and help reduce bloating and gas, increase energy, and maintain proper glucose and insulin levels). Feel free to use whatever you like.

Day 1 Sunday*

The first thing to do upon waking up is to drink 16 ounces of water. Here, as in all my meal plans, I focus on hydration right away in the morning.

Meal 1: Spinach Shake
(about 400 calories)
Multivitamin
Digestive enzymes

Meal 2: Midmorning snack
(about 200 calories)
1 handful blueberries,
1 large handful almonds

Meal 3: Spinach Shake
(about 400 calories)
Digestive enzymes

Meal 4: Midafternoon snack
(about 300 calories)
1 banana with 2 tablespoons natural peanut butter, 1 handful raspberries

Meal 5: Sun-Dried Tomato Chicken
(about 400 calories)**
Add 2 cups steamed asparagus on the side.
Digestive enzymes

---

* Though we start the meal plan on Sunday, you can of course start any day of the week. The meal plan is outlined to cook a bulk of your meats in advance on Sunday and then again midweek on Wednesday. Feel free to adjust as needed.

** Make enough of this recipe to last for three meals and refrigerate leftovers in tightly sealed containers for use later in the week.

Day 2 Monday

Drink 16 ounces water.

Meal 1: Spinach Shake
(about 400 calories)
Multivitamin
Digestive enzymes

Meal 2: Midmorning snack
(about 200 calories)
1 handful blueberries,
1 large handful almonds

Meal 3: Sun-Dried Tomato Chicken
(about 400 calories)
Add 2 cups steamed asparagus on the side.
Digestive enzymes

Meal 4: Midafternoon snack
(about 200 calories)
1 large handful pumpkin seeds,
1 handful raspberries

Meal 5: Citrus Salmon with Avocado Salsa (about 450 calories)
Digestive enzymes

Day 3 Tuesday

Drink 16 ounces water.

Meal 1: Egg-White Breakfast Burrito without the tortilla (about 450 calories)
Multivitamin
Digestive enzymes

Meal 2: Midmorning snack (about 250 calories)
1 handful blueberries, 1 handful strawberries, 1 large handful almonds

Meal 3: Sun-Dried Tomato Chicken on a salad (about 450 calories)
Place 1 cup leftover Sun-Dried Tomato Chicken, ¼ cup chopped red and yellow bell peppers, ¼ cup chopped cucumbers, and 1 handful almonds on top of a mixed dark green salad with an oil-based vinaigrette dressing.
Digestive enzymes

Meal 4: Midafternoon snack (about 300 calories)
1 handful strawberries, 1 handful pumpkin seeds, 1 low-sugar, high-fiber protein bar (preferably with a ratio of 1g fiber/1g protein, but no less than .5g/1g)

Meal 5: Spinach Shake (about 400 calories)
Digestive enzymes

Day 4 Wednesday

Drink 16 ounces water.

Meal 1: Spinach Shake (about 400 calories)
Multivitamin
Digestive enzymes

Meal 2: Midmorning snack (about 350 calories)
1 banana with 2 tablespoons natural peanut butter, 1 handful roasted pecans

Meal 3: Turkey Breast and Berry Salad (about 400 calories)
Digestive enzymes

Meal 4: Midafternoon snack (about 250 calories)
1 handful beef jerky,
1 large handful cashews

Meal 5: Beef Fajitas (about 450 calories)*
Add 2 cups steamed yellow squash.
Digestive enzymes

---

* Make enough of this recipe to last for three meals and refrigerate leftovers in tightly sealed containers for use later in the week.

Day 5 Thursday

Drink 16 ounces water.

Meal 1: Spinach Egg-White Omelet
(about 400 calories)
Multivitamin
Digestive enzymes

Meal 2: Midmorning snack
(about 200 calories)
1 handful strawberries,
1 large handful beef jerky

Meal 3: Beef Fajitas
(about 450 calories)
Add 2 cups steamed yellow squash.
Digestive enzymes

Meal 4: Midafternoon snack
(about 250 calories)
1 handful blueberries, 1 handful raspberries, 1 large handful almonds

Meal 5: Turkey Breast and Berry Salad (about 400 calories)
Digestive enzymes

Day 6 Friday

Drink 16 ounces water.

Meal 1: Spinach Shake
(about 400 calories)
Multivitamin
Digestive enzymes

Meal 2: Midmorning snack
(about 200 calories)
1 handful blueberries, 1 low-sugar, high-fiber protein bar (preferably with a ratio of 1g fiber/1g protein, but no less than .5g/1g)

Meal 3: Beef Fajitas on a salad
(about 450 calories)
Place 1 cup leftover Beef Fajitas meat, 1 sliced red pepper, and 1 handful roasted pecans on a mixed dark green salad with an oil-based vinaigrette dressing.
Digestive enzymes

Meal 4: Midafternoon snack
(about 200 calories)
1 handful almonds, 1 handful strawberries, 1 handful raspberries

Meal 5: Sea Salt Salmon with Olive Oil Mayo (about 450 calories)
Add 2 cups steamed broccoli on the side.
Digestive enzymes

Day 7 Saturday

Drink 16 ounces water.

Meal 1: Spinach Shake
(about 400 calories)
Multivitamin
Digestive enzymes

Meal 2: Midmorning snack
(about 250 calories)
1 large handful almonds,
1 handful beef jerky

Meal 3: Spinach Egg-White Omelet
(about 400 calories)
Digestive enzymes

Meal 4: Midafternoon snack
(about 300 calories)
1 handful strawberries, 1 large handful pumpkin seeds, 1 handful beef jerky

Meal 5: Spinach Shake
(about 400 calories)
Digestive enzymes

Day 8 Sunday

Drink 16 ounces water.

Meal 1: Spinach Shake
(about 400 calories)
Multivitamin
Digestive enzymes

Meal 2: Midmorning snack
(about 250 calories)
1 handful pumpkin seeds, 1 low-sugar, high-fiber protein bar (preferably with a ratio of 1g fiber/1g protein, but no less than .5g/1g)

Meal 3: Spinach Egg-White Omelet
(about 400 calories)
Digestive enzymes

Meal 4: Midafternoon snack
(about 200 calories)
1 handful blueberries, 1 handful raspberries, 1 handful almonds

Meal 5: Roast Chicken
(about 450 calories)*
Add 2 cups steamed cauliflower on the side.
Digestive enzymes

---

* Make enough of this recipe to last for three meals and refrigerate leftovers in tightly sealed containers for use later in the week.

Day 9 Monday

Drink 16 ounces water.

Meal 1: Spinach Shake
(about 400 calories)
Multivitamin
Digestive enzymes

Meal 2: Midmorning snack
(about 350 calories)
1 banana with 2 tablespoons natural peanut butter, 1 handful almonds

Meal 3: Roast Chicken
(about 450 calories)
Add 2 cups steamed cauliflower on the side.
Digestive enzymes

Meal 4: Midafternoon snack
(about 200 calories)
1 large handful pumpkin seeds, 1 handful blueberries

Meal 5: Caramelized Onion–Glazed Salmon (about 450 calories)
Add 2 cups steamed green beans on the side.
Digestive enzymes

Day 10 Tuesday

Drink 16 ounces water.

Meal 1: Egg-White Breakfast Burrito without the tortilla
(about 450 calories)
Multivitamin
Digestive enzymes

Meal 2: Midmorning snack
(about 250 calories)
1 grapefruit, 1 low-sugar, high-fiber protein bar (preferably with a ratio of 1g fiber/1g protein, but no less than .5g/1g)

Meal 3: Roast Chicken on a salad
(about 450 calories)
Place 1 leftover Roast Chicken breast with 1 cup leftover peppers on a mixed dark green salad with an oil-based vinaigrette dressing.
Digestive enzymes

Meal 4: Midafternoon snack
(about 250 calories)
1 handful beef jerky, 1 handful pumpkin seeds, 1 handful strawberries

Meal 5: Spinach Shake
(about 400 calories)
Digestive enzymes

Day 11 Wednesday

Drink 16 ounces water.

Meal 1: Spinach Shake
(about 400 calories)
Multivitamin
Digestive enzymes

Meal 2: Midmorning snack
(about 200 calories)
1 handful blueberries,
1 large handful roasted pecans

Meal 3: Turkey Breast and Berry Salad (about 400 calories)
Digestive enzymes

Meal 4: Midafternoon snack
(about 300 calories)
1 large handful pumpkin seeds,
1 handful almonds, 1 handful raspberries

Meal 5: Turkey Fajitas (substitute turkey breast for beef in the Beef Fajitas recipe) (about 450 calories)*
Add 2 cups steamed zucchini on the side.
Digestive enzymes

---

* Make enough of this recipe to last for three meals and refrigerate leftovers in tightly sealed containers for use later in the week.

Day 12 Thursday

Drink 16 ounces water.

Meal 1: Spinach Shake
(about 400 calories)
Multivitamin
Digestive enzymes

Meal 2: Midmorning snack
(about 300 calories)
1 handful almonds, 1 handful strawberries, 1 low-sugar, high-fiber protein bar (preferably with a ratio of 1g fiber/1g protein, but no less than .5g/1g)

Meal 3: Turkey Fajitas
(about 450 calories)
Add 2 cups steamed zucchini on the side.
Digestive enzymes

Meal 4: Midafternoon snack
(about 300 calories)
Celery with 2 tablespoons natural peanut butter, 1 handful cashews

Meal 5: Spinach Egg-White Omelet
(about 400 calories)
Digestive enzymes

Day 13 Friday

Drink 16 ounces water.

Meal 1: Spinach Shake
(about 400 calories)
Multivitamin
Digestive enzymes

Meal 2: Midmorning snack
(about 200 calories)
1 handful almonds, 1 handful strawberries, 1 handful blueberries

Meal 3: Turkey Fajitas on a salad
(about 500 calories)
Place 1 cup leftover Turkey Fajitas meat, 1 sliced pepper (your choice), and ¼ cup sliced avocado on a mixed dark green salad with an oil-based vinaigrette dressing.
Digestive enzymes

Meal 4: Midafternoon snack
(about 300 calories)
Celery with 2 tablespoons natural peanut butter, 1 handful pumpkin seeds

Meal 5: Citrus Salmon with Avocado Salsa (about 450 calories)
Add 2 cups steamed broccoli on the side.
Digestive enzymes

Day 14 Saturday

Drink 16 ounces water.

Meal 1: Spinach Shake
(about 400 calories)
Multivitamin
Digestive enzymes

Meal 2: Midmorning snack
(about 250 calories)
1 handful almonds, 1 handful beef jerky, 1 small handful blueberries

Meal 3: Spinach Egg-White Omelet
(about 400 calories)
Digestive enzymes

Meal 4: Midafternoon snack
(about 200 calories)
1 handful raspberries,
1 large handful pumpkin seeds

Meal 5: Citrus Salmon with Avocado Salsa on a salad (about 450 calories)
Place 1 fillet of leftover Citrus Salmon on a mixed dark green salad with leftover Avocado Salsa.
Digestive enzymes

Day 15 Sunday

Drink 16 ounces water.

Meal 1: Spinach Shake
(about 400 calories)
Multivitamin
Digestive enzymes

Meal 2: Midmorning snack
(about 300 calories)
1 handful pumpkin seeds, 1 handful strawberries, 1 low-sugar, high-fiber protein bar (preferably with a ratio of 1g fiber/1g protein, but no less than .5g/1g)

Meal 3: Egg-White Breakfast Burrito without the tortilla (about 450 calories)
Digestive enzymes

Meal 4: Midafternoon snack
(about 250 calories)
1 handful almonds, 1 handful beef jerky, 1 handful blueberries

Meal 5: Mexican Chicken
(about 450 calories; leave out the cheese in this recipe for this month)*
Add 2 cups steamed cauliflower on the side.
Digestive enzymes

* Make enough of this recipe to last for three meals and refrigerate leftovers in tightly sealed containers for use later in the week.

Day 16 Monday

Drink 16 ounces water.

Meal 1: Spinach Shake
(about 400 calories)
Multivitamin
Digestive enzymes

Meal 2: Midmorning snack
(about 200 calories)
1 handful raspberries,
1 large handful almonds

Meal 3: Mexican Chicken
(about 450 calories)
Add 2 cups steamed cauliflower on the side.
Digestive enzymes

Meal 4: Midafternoon snack
(about 350 calories)
1 banana with 2 tablespoons natural peanut butter, 1 handful pumpkin seeds

Meal 5: Sea Salt Salmon with Olive Oil Mayo (about 450 calories)
Add 2 cups steamed asparagus on the side.
Digestive enzymes

Day 17 Tuesday

Drink 16 ounces water.

Meal 1: Egg-White Breakfast Burrito without the tortilla (about 450 calories)
Multivitamin
Digestive enzymes

Meal 2: Midmorning snack (about 250 calories)
1 handful blueberries, 1 handful roasted pecans, 1 handful beef jerky

Meal 3: Mexican Chicken on a salad (about 450 calories)
Place 1 cup leftover Mexican Chicken, ¼ cup sliced avocado, and ¼ cup sliced yellow pepper on a mixed dark green salad with an oil-based vinaigrette dressing.
Digestive enzymes

Meal 4: Midafternoon snack (about 250 calories)
1 handful almonds, 1 low-sugar, high-fiber protein bar (preferably with a ratio of 1g fiber/1g protein, but no less than .5g/1g)

Meal 5: Spinach Shake (about 400 calories)
Digestive enzymes

Day 18 Wednesday

Drink 16 ounces water.

Meal 1: Spinach Shake (about 400 calories)
Multivitamin
Digestive enzymes

Meal 2: Midmorning snack (about 200 calories)
1 handful blueberries,
1 large handful almonds

Meal 3: Turkey Breast and Berry Salad (about 400 calories)
Digestive enzymes

Meal 4: Midafternoon snack (about 250 calories)
1 handful blueberries, 1 handful raspberries, 1 large handful roasted pecans

Meal 5: Sun-Dried Tomato Chicken (about 400 calories)*
Add 2 cups steamed green beans on the side.
Digestive enzymes

---

* Make enough of this recipe to last for three meals and refrigerate leftovers in tightly sealed containers for use later in the week.

Day 19 Thursday

Drink 16 ounces water.

Meal 1: Spinach Shake
(about 400 calories)
Multivitamin
Digestive enzymes

Meal 2: Midmorning snack
(about 250 calories)
1 handful blueberries, 1 handful almonds, 1 handful beef jerky

Meal 3: Sun-Dried Tomato Chicken
(about 400 calories)
Add 1 cup steamed red peppers and 1 cup steamed cauliflower on the side.
Digestive enzymes

Meal 4: Midafternoon snack
(about 200 calories)
1 handful strawberries, 1 low-sugar, high-fiber protein bar (preferably with a ratio of 1g fiber/1g protein, but no less than .5g/1g)

Meal 5: Spinach Egg-White Omelet
(about 400 calories)
Digestive enzymes

Day 20 Friday

Drink 16 ounces water.

Meal 1: Spinach Shake
(about 400 calories)
Multivitamin
Digestive enzymes

Meal 2: Midmorning snack
(about 350 calories)
1 banana with 2 tablespoons natural peanut butter, 1 large handful almonds

Meal 3: Sun-Dried Tomato Chicken on a salad (about 450 calories)
Place ½ cup leftover Sun-Dried Tomato Chicken, 1 small handful cashews, 1 handful blueberries, and 1 handful strawberries on a mixed dark green salad with a low-calorie vinaigrette dressing. (Raspberry vinaigrette goes well with berry salads.)
Digestive enzymes

Meal 4: Midafternoon snack
(about 250 calories)
1 large handful roasted pecans, 1 handful beef jerky

Meal 5: Caramelized Onion–Glazed Salmon (about 450 calories)
Add 2 cups steamed zucchini on the side.
Digestive enzymes

Day 21 Saturday

Drink 16 ounces water.

Meal 1: Egg-White Breakfast Burrito without the tortilla (about 450 calories)
Multivitamin
Digestive enzymes

Meal 2: Midmorning snack (about 300 calories)
Celery with 2 tablespoons natural peanut butter, 1 handful beef jerky

Meal 3: Caramelized Onion–Glazed Salmon on a salad (about 500 calories)
Place 1 leftover fillet of Caramelized Onion–Glazed Salmon on a mixed dark green salad with an oil-based vinaigrette dressing.
Digestive enzymes

Meal 4: Midafternoon snack (about 200 calories)
1 handful blueberries,
1 large handful pumpkin seeds

Meal 5: Spinach Shake (about 400 calories)
Digestive enzymes

Day 22 Sunday

Drink 16 ounces water.

Meal 1: Spinach Egg-White Omelet (about 400 calories)
Multivitamin
Digestive enzymes

Meal 2: Midmorning snack (about 300 calories)
1 handful blueberries, 1 handful almonds, 1 low-sugar, high-fiber protein bar (preferably with a ratio of 1g fiber/1g protein, but no less than .5g/1g)

Meal 3: Spinach Shake (about 400 calories)
Digestive enzymes

Meal 4: Midafternoon snack (about 300 calories)
Celery with 2 tablespoons natural peanut butter, 1 handful beef jerky

Meal 5: BBQ Chicken Lettuce Wraps (about 450 calories)*
Add 2 cups steamed yellow squash on the side.
Digestive enzymes

---

* Make enough of this recipe to last for three meals and refrigerate leftovers in tightly sealed containers for use later in the week.

Day 23 Monday

Drink 16 ounces water.

Meal 1: Spinach Shake
(about 400 calories)
Multivitamin
Digestive enzymes

Meal 2: Midmorning snack
(about 200 calories)
1 handful blueberries, 1 low-sugar, high-fiber protein bar (preferably with a ratio of 1g fiber/1g protein, but no less than .5g/1g)

Meal 3: BBQ Chicken Lettuce Wraps
(about 450 calories)
Add 2 cups steamed yellow squash on the side.
Digestive enzymes

Meal 4: Midafternoon snack
(about 250 calories)
1 handful cashews, 1 handful beef jerky, 1 handful raspberries

Meal 5: Sea Salt Salmon with Olive Oil Mayo (about 450 calories)
Add 2 cups steamed green beans on the side.
Digestive enzymes

Day 24 Tuesday

Drink 16 ounces water.

Meal 1: Spinach Shake
(about 400 calories)
Multivitamin
Digestive enzymes

Meal 2: Midmorning snack
(about 300 calories)
Celery with 2 tablespoons natural peanut butter, 1 handful almonds

Meal 3: BBQ Chicken Lettuce Wraps on a salad (about 450 calories)
Place 1 cup leftover BBQ Chicken and ¼ cup chopped red onion on a mixed dark green salad with an oil-based vinaigrette dressing.
Digestive enzymes

Meal 4: Midafternoon snack
(about 300 calories)
1 handful beef jerky, 1 large handful pumpkin seeds, 1 handful blueberries

Meal 5: Spinach Egg-White Omelet
(about 400 calories)
Digestive enzymes

Day 25 Wednesday

Drink 16 ounces water.

Meal 1: Spinach Shake
(about 400 calories)
Multivitamin
Digestive enzymes

Meal 2: Midmorning snack
(about 250 calories)
1 handful pumpkin seeds, 1 handful almonds, 1 handful raspberries

Meal 3: Turkey Breast and Berry Salad (about 400 calories)
Digestive enzymes

Meal 4: Midafternoon snack
(about 350 calories)
1 banana with 2 tablespoons natural peanut butter, 1 handful beef jerky

Meal 5: Basil Chicken with Vegetables (about 450 calories)*
Digestive enzymes

* Make enough of this recipe to last for three meals and refrigerate leftovers in tightly sealed containers for use later in the week.

Day 26 Thursday

Drink 16 ounces water.

Meal 1: Spinach Egg-White Omelet
(about 400 calories)
Multivitamin
Digestive enzymes

Meal 2: Midmorning snack
(about 300 calories)
1 large handful almonds, 1 handful beef jerky, 1 handful blueberries

Meal 3: Basil Chicken with Vegetables (about 450 calories)
Digestive enzymes

Meal 4: Midafternoon snack
(about 300 calories)
1 handful pumpkin seeds, 1 handful blueberries, 1 low-sugar, high-fiber protein bar (preferably with a ratio of 1g fiber/1g protein, but no less than .5g/1g)

Meal 5: Spinach Shake
(about 400 calories)
Digestive enzymes

Day 27 Friday

Drink 16 ounces water.

Meal 1: Spinach Shake
(about 400 calories)
Multivitamin
Digestive enzymes

Meal 2: Midmorning snack
(about 250 calories)
1 handful raspberries, 1 handful beef jerky, 1 handful pumpkin seeds

Meal 3: Basil Chicken with Vegetables (about 450 calories)
Digestive enzymes

Meal 4: Midafternoon snack
(about 250 calories)
1 large handful almonds,
1 small handful beef jerky

Meal 5: Citrus Salmon with Avocado Salsa (about 450 calories)
Add 2 cups steamed green beans on the side.
Digestive enzymes

Day 28 Saturday

Drink 16 ounces water.

Meal 1: Spinach Egg-White Omelet
(about 400 calories)
Multivitamin
Digestive enzymes

Meal 2: Midmorning snack
(about 300 calories)
Celery with 2 tablespoons natural peanut butter, 1 handful roasted pecans

Meal 3: Spinach Shake
(about 400 calories)
Digestive enzymes

Meal 4: Midafternoon snack
(about 250 calories)
1 handful blueberries, 1 handful strawberries, 1 large handful almonds

Meal 5: Citrus Salmon with Avocado Salsa on a salad (about 450 calories)
Place 1 fillet of leftover Citrus Salmon on a mixed dark green salad with leftover Avocado Salsa.
Digestive enzymes

Meal Plan 2: The Balance

The following monthlong meal plan is designed specifically for when you've started to really integrate healthy eating and workouts into your daily routine. This meal plan is extremely balanced and sustainable. I used a version of this for months 2 through 4 on my journey from Fat2Fit. I also reintegrated this meal plan once I hit my goal of 193 pounds after my Fat2Fit stage was complete. The results were fantastic, and I am confident that these guidelines can work for you.

Remember that I believe people should eat approximately every three hours throughout the day. Obviously, schedules for all of us are different, but the goal is to achieve a balanced regimen. Do what you can to fit these meals in.

Because this plan is based on a man's caloric needs, I recommend that women reduce the overall daily caloric intake by 500 calories (a greater reduction than in the previous meal plan), again either by reducing portion size or by omitting certain foods or meals. Also, you'll notice that I built two cheat/treat meals into this month's meal plan. In months 2 through 4 of my Fat2Fit journey, I had only two cheat meals per month, but once I reached my goal I loosened up: I now usually build in one cheat meal per week. You can adjust the cheat meals based on your own needs.

Day 1 Sunday*

The first thing to do upon waking up is to drink 16 ounces of water. As with all of my meal plans, I focus on hydration right away in the morning.

Meal 1: Farmer's Breakfast Scramble (about 550 calories)
Multivitamin
Digestive enzymes

Meal 2: Midmorning snack (about 300 calories)
1 handful blueberries, 1 handful almonds, 1 low-sugar, high-fiber protein bar (preferably with a ratio of 1g fiber/1g protein, but no less than .5g/1g)

Meal 3: Spinach Shake (about 400 calories)
Digestive enzymes

Meal 4: Midafternoon snack (about 250 calories)
Celery with 2 tablespoons natural peanut butter, 1 handful raspberries,

Meal 5: Chinese "Fried Rice" (about 450 calories)**
Digestive enzymes

---

* Though we start the meal plan on Sunday, you can of course start any day of the week. The meal plan is outlined to cook a bulk of your meats in advance on Sunday and then again midweek on Wednesday. Feel free to adjust as needed.

** Make enough of this recipe to last for three meals and refrigerate leftovers in tightly sealed containers for use later in the week.

Day 2 Monday

Drink 16 ounces water.

Meal 1: Pumpkin Pie Protein Shake (about 300 calories)
Multivitamin
Digestive enzymes

Meal 2: Midmorning snack (about 350 calories)
1 banana with 2 tablespoons natural peanut butter, 1 handful almonds

Meal 3: Chinese "Fried Rice" (about 450 calories)
Digestive enzymes

Meal 4: Midafternoon snack (about 250 calories)
1 apple, 1 handful pumpkin seeds, 1 handful beef jerky

Meal 5: Caramelized Onion–Glazed Salmon (about 450 calories)
Add 1 cup steamed zucchini on the side.
Digestive enzymes

Meal 6: Pre/Postworkout snack (about 300 calories)
1 slice whole-wheat toast with 1 tablespoon peanut butter and ¼ protein shake (1 scoop vanilla whey protein with water only) 45 to 30 minutes before workout, and the other ¾ protein shake after workout

Day 3 Tuesday

Drink 16 ounces water.

Meal 1: Farmer's Breakfast Scramble (about 550 calories)
Multivitamin
Digestive enzymes

Meal 2: Midmorning snack (about 200 calories)
1 handful blueberries, 1 handful strawberries, 1 handful almonds

Meal 3: Chinese "Fried Rice" (about 450 calories)
Digestive enzymes

Meal 4: Midafternoon snack (about 250 calories)
1 apple, 1 handful beef jerky, 1 handful almonds

Meal 5: Spinach Shake (about 400 calories)
Digestive enzymes

Meal 6: Pre/Postworkout snack (about 250 calories)
1 banana with 1 tablespoon peanut butter and ¼ protein shake (1 scoop vanilla whey protein with water only) 45 to 30 minutes before workout, and the other ¾ protein shake after workout

Day 4 Wednesday

Drink 16 ounces water.

Meal 1: Spinach Shake (about 400 calories)
Multivitamin
Digestive enzymes

Meal 2: Midmorning snack (about 300 calories)
1 handful raspberries, 1 handful pumpkin seeds, 1 low-sugar, high-fiber protein bar (preferably with a ratio of 1g fiber/1g protein, but no less than .5g/1g)

Meal 3: Turkey Breast and Berry Salad (about 400 calories)
Digestive enzymes

Meal 4: Midafternoon snack (about 250 calories)
1 grapefruit, 1 handful baby carrots, 1 handful beef jerky

Meal 5: Mexican Chicken (about 450 calories)*
Add 1 cup steamed asparagus on the side.
Digestive enzymes

Meal 6: Pre/Postworkout snack (about 300 calories)
1 slice whole-wheat toast with 1 tablespoon peanut butter and ¼ protein shake (1 scoop vanilla whey protein with water only) 45 to 30 minutes before workout, and the other ¾ protein shake after workout

---

* Make enough of this recipe to last for three meals and refrigerate leftovers in tightly sealed containers for use later in the week.

Day 5 Thursday

Drink 16 ounces water.

Meal 1: Spinach Egg-White Omelet (about 400 calories)
Multivitamin
Digestive enzymes

Meal 2: Midmorning snack (about 250 calories)
1 grapefruit, 1 handful baby carrots, 1 handful almonds

Meal 3: Mexican Chicken (about 450 calories)
Digestive enzymes

Meal 4: Midafternoon snack (about 250 calories)
Celery with 2 tablespoons natural peanut butter, 1 apple

Meal 5: Turkey Breast and Berry Salad (about 400 calories)
Digestive enzymes

Meal 6: Pre/Postworkout snack (about 250 calories)
1 banana with 1 tablespoon peanut butter and ¼ protein shake (1 scoop vanilla whey protein with water only) 45 to 30 minutes before workout, and the other ¾ protein shake after workout

Day 6 Friday

Drink 16 ounces water.

Meal 1: Pumpkin Pie Protein Shake (about 300 calories)
Multivitamin
Digestive enzymes

Meal 2: Midmorning snack (about 250 calories)
1 handful almonds, 1 handful raspberries, 1 grapefruit

Meal 3: Mexican Chicken on a salad (about 450 calories)
Place 1 cup leftover Mexican Chicken, ¼ cup sliced red pepper, and ¼ cup sliced avocado on a mixed dark green salad with an oil-based vinaigrette dressing.
Digestive enzymes

Meal 4: Midafternoon snack (about 300 calories)
1 handful pumpkin seeds, 1 handful blueberries, 1 low-sugar, high-fiber protein bar (preferably with a ratio of 1g fiber/1g protein, but no less than .5g/1g)

Meal 5: Citrus Salmon with Avocado Salsa (about 450 calories)
Add 1 cup steamed broccoli on the side.
Digestive enzymes

Meal 6: Pre/Postworkout snack (about 300 calories)
1 slice whole-wheat toast with 1 tablespoon peanut butter and ¼ protein shake (1 scoop vanilla whey protein with water only) 45 to 30 minutes before workout, and the other ¾ protein shake after workout

Day 7 Saturday

Drink 16 ounces water.

Meal 1: Spinach Shake
(about 400 calories)
Multivitamin
Digestive enzymes

Meal 2: Midmorning snack
(about 250 calories)
1 handful almonds, 1 handful beef jerky, 1 small handful raspberries

Meal 3: Spinach Egg-White Omelet
(about 400 calories)
Digestive enzymes

Meal 4: Midafternoon snack
(about 350 calories)
1 banana with 2 tablespoons natural peanut butter, 1 small handful pumpkin seeds

Meal 5: ★Cheat/Treat Meal★
(about 700 calories)
Eat whatever you want as long as your other four meals today were nutritious, but try to keep it under 700 calories.
Digestive enzymes

Day 8 Sunday

Drink 16 ounces water.

Meal 1: Spinach Shake
(about 400 calories)
Multivitamin
Digestive enzymes

Meal 2: Midmorning snack
(about 250 calories)
1 handful pumpkin seeds, 1 low-sugar, high-fiber protein bar (preferably with a ratio of 1g fiber/1g protein, but no less than .5g/1g)

Meal 3: Egg-White Breakfast Burrito
(about 500 calories)
Digestive enzymes

Meal 4: Midafternoon snack
(about 250 calories)
1 handful blueberries, 1 handful almonds, 1 handful beef jerky

Meal 5: BBQ Chicken Lettuce Wraps
(about 450 calories)*
Add 1 cup steamed cauliflower on the side.
Digestive enzymes

---

* Make enough of this recipe to last for three meals and refrigerate leftovers in tightly sealed containers for use later in the week.

Day 9 Monday

Drink 16 ounces water.

Meal 1: Pumpkin Pie Protein Shake (about 300 calories)
Multivitamin
Digestive enzymes

Meal 2: Midmorning snack (about 350 calories)
1 banana with 2 tablespoons natural peanut butter, 1 handful almonds

Meal 3: BBQ Chicken Lettuce Wraps on a salad (about 500 calories)
Place 1 cup leftover BBQ Chicken and ¼ cup chopped red pepper on a mixed dark green salad with an oil-based vinaigrette dressing.
Digestive enzymes

Meal 4: Midafternoon snack (about 250 calories)
1 handful raspberries, 1 handful strawberries, 1 large handful pumpkin seeds

Meal 5: Sea Salt Salmon with Olive Oil Mayo (about 450 calories)
Add 1 cup steamed asparagus on the side.
Digestive enzymes

Meal 6: Pre/Postworkout snack (about 300 calories)
1 slice whole-wheat toast with 1 tablespoon peanut butter and ¼ protein shake (1 scoop vanilla whey protein with water only) 45 to 30 minutes before workout, and the other ¾ protein shake after workout

Day 10 Tuesday

Drink 16 ounces water.

Meal 1: Egg-White Breakfast Burrito (about 500 calories)
Multivitamin
Digestive enzymes

Meal 2: Midmorning snack (about 300 calories)
1 grapefruit, 1 handful baby carrots, 1 low-sugar, high-fiber protein bar (preferably with a ratio of 1g fiber/1g protein, but no less than .5g/1g)

Meal 3: BBQ Chicken Lettuce Wraps (about 450 calories)
Add 1 cup steamed asparagus on the side.
Digestive enzymes

Meal 4: Midafternoon snack (about 300 calories)
1 apple, 1 handful beef jerky, 1 large handful pumpkin seeds

Meal 5: Spinach Shake (about 400 calories)
Digestive enzymes

Meal 6: Pre/Postworkout snack (about 250 calories)
1 banana with 1 tablespoon peanut butter and ¼ protein shake (1 scoop vanilla whey protein with water only) 45 to 30 minutes before workout, and the other ¾ protein shake after workout

Day 11 Wednesday

Drink 16 ounces water.

Meal 1: Pumpkin Pie Protein Shake (about 300 calories)
Multivitamin
Digestive enzymes

Meal 2: Midmorning snack (about 300 calories)
1 banana with 2 tablespoons natural peanut butter, 1 handful blueberries

Meal 3: Turkey Breast and Berry Salad (about 400 calories)
Digestive enzymes

Meal 4: Midafternoon snack (about 200 calories)
1 handful pumpkin seeds,
1 handful beef jerky

Meal 5: Beef Fajitas with 1 low-carb tortilla (about 550 calories)*
Digestive enzymes

Meal 6: Pre/Postworkout snack (about 300 calories)
1 slice whole-wheat toast with 1 tablespoon peanut butter and ¼ protein shake (1 scoop vanilla whey protein with water only) 45 to 30 minutes before workout, and the other ¾ protein shake after workout

---

* Make enough of this recipe to last for three meals and refrigerate leftovers in tightly sealed containers for use later in the week.

Day 12 Thursday

Drink 16 ounces water.

Meal 1: Spinach Shake (about 400 calories)
Multivitamin
Digestive enzymes

Meal 2: Midmorning snack (about 300 calories)
1 handful almonds, 1 handful strawberries, 1 low-sugar, high-fiber protein bar (preferably with a ratio of 1g fiber/1g protein, but no less than .5g/1g)

Meal 3: Beef Fajitas (about 450 calories)
Add 1 cup steamed yellow squash
Digestive enzymes

Meal 4: Midafternoon snack (about 300 calories)
1 grapefruit, celery with
2 tablespoons natural peanut butter

Meal 5: Spinach Egg-White Omelet (about 400 calories)
Digestive enzymes

Meal 6: Pre/Postworkout snack (about 250 calories)
1 banana with 1 tablespoon peanut butter and ¼ protein shake (1 scoop vanilla whey protein with water only) 45 to 30 minutes before workout, and the other ¾ protein shake after workout

Day 13 Friday

Drink 16 ounces water.

Meal 1: Pumpkin Pie Protein Shake (about 300 calories)
Multivitamin
Digestive enzymes

Meal 2: Midmorning snack (about 300 calories)
1 handful almonds, 1 handful strawberries, 1 low-sugar, high-fiber protein bar (preferably with a ratio of 1g fiber/1g protein, but no less than .5g/1g)

Meal 3: Beef Fajitas on a salad (about 450 calories)
Place 1 cup leftover Beef Fajitas meat and 1 sliced pepper (your choice) on a mixed dark green salad with an oil-based vinaigrette dressing.
Digestive enzymes

Meal 4: Midafternoon snack (about 200 calories)
1 apple, 1 handful pumpkin seeds, 1 handful baby carrots

Meal 5: Caramelized Onion–Glazed Salmon (about 450 calories)
Add 1 cup steamed broccoli on the side.
Digestive enzymes

Meal 6: Pre/Postworkout snack (about 300 calories)
1 slice whole-wheat toast with 1 tablespoon peanut butter and ¼ protein shake (1 scoop vanilla whey protein with water only) 45 to 30 minutes before workout, and the other ¾ protein shake after workout

Day 14 Saturday

Drink 16 ounces water.

Meal 1: Spinach Shake (about 400 calories)
Multivitamin
Digestive enzymes

Meal 2: Midmorning snack (about 300 calories)
1 large handful almonds, 1 handful beef jerky, 1 small handful blueberries

Meal 3: Farmer's Breakfast Scramble (about 550 calories)
Digestive enzymes

Meal 4: Midafternoon snack (about 350 calories)
1 banana with 2 tablespoons natural peanut butter, 1 handful pumpkin seeds

Meal 5: Caramelized Onion–Glazed Salmon (about 450 calories)
Place 1 fillet of leftover Caramelized Onion–Glazed Salmon on a mixed dark green salad with an oil-based vinaigrette dressing.
Digestive enzymes

Day 15 Sunday

Drink 16 ounces water.

Meal 1: Spinach Shake
(about 400 calories)
Multivitamin
Digestive enzymes

Meal 2: Midmorning snack
(about 300 calories)
1 handful pumpkin seeds, 1 apple, 1 low-sugar, high-fiber protein bar (preferably with a ratio of 1g fiber/1g protein, but no less than .5g/1g)

Meal 3: Farmer's Breakfast Scramble
(about 550 calories)
Digestive enzymes

Meal 4: Midafternoon snack
(about 250 calories)
1 banana with 2 tablespoons natural peanut butter

Meal 5: Roast Chicken
(about 450 calories)*
Digestive enzymes

---

* Make enough of this recipe to last for three meals and refrigerate leftovers in tightly sealed containers for use later in the week.

Day 16 Monday

Drink 16 ounces water.

Meal 1: Spinach Shake
(about 400 calories)
Multivitamin
Digestive enzymes

Meal 2: Midmorning snack
(about 350 calories)
1 banana with 2 tablespoons natural peanut butter, 1 handful almonds

Meal 3: Roast Chicken
(about 450 calories)
Digestive enzymes

Meal 4: Midafternoon snack
(about 250 calories)
1 grapefruit, 1 handful raspberries, 1 handful pumpkin seeds

Meal 5: Sea Salt Salmon with Olive Oil Mayo (about 450 calories)
Add 1 cup steamed asparagus on the side.
Digestive enzymes

Meal 6: Pre/Postworkout snack
(about 300 calories)
1 slice whole-wheat toast with 1 tablespoon peanut butter and ¼ protein shake (1 scoop vanilla whey protein with water only) 45 to 30 minutes before workout, and the other ¾ protein shake after workout

Day 17 Tuesday

Drink 16 ounces water.

Meal 1: Egg-White Breakfast Burrito (about 500 calories)
Multivitamin
Digestive enzymes

Meal 2: Midmorning snack (about 250 calories)
1 handful blueberries, 1 handful roasted pecans, 1 handful beef jerky

Meal 3: Roast Chicken on a salad (about 500 calories)
Place 1 leftover Roast Chicken breast and 1 cup leftover roasted red peppers on a mixed dark green salad with an oil-based vinaigrette dressing.
Digestive enzymes

Meal 4: Midafternoon snack (about 300 calories)
1 grapefruit, 1 handful baby carrots, 1 low-sugar, high-fiber protein bar (preferably with a ratio of 1g fiber/1g protein, but no less than .5g/1g)

Meal 5: Spinach Shake (about 400 calories)
Digestive enzymes

Meal 6: Pre/Postworkout snack (about 250 calories)
1 banana with 1 tablespoon peanut butter and ¼ protein shake (1 scoop vanilla whey protein with water only) 45 to 30 minutes before workout, and the other ¾ protein shake after workout

Day 18 Wednesday

Drink 16 ounces water.

Meal 1: Pumpkin Pie Protein Shake (about 300 calories)
Multivitamin
Digestive enzymes

Meal 2: Midmorning snack (about 200 calories)
1 handful blueberries, 1 large handful almonds

Meal 3: Turkey Breast and Berry Salad (about 400 calories)
Digestive enzymes

Meal 4: Midafternoon snack (about 300 calories)
Celery with 2 tablespoons natural peanut butter, 1 handful roasted pecans

Meal 5: Sun-Dried Tomato Chicken (about 400 calories)*
Add 1 cup steamed green beans on the side.
Digestive enzymes

Meal 6: Pre/Postworkout snack (about 300 calories)
1 slice whole-wheat toast with 1 tablespoon peanut butter and ¼ protein shake (1 scoop vanilla whey protein with water only) 45 to 30 minutes before workout, and the other ¾ protein shake after workout

---

* Make enough of this recipe to last for three meals and refrigerate leftovers in tightly sealed containers for use later in the week.

Day 19 Thursday

Drink 16 ounces water.

Meal 1: Spinach Shake
(about 400 calories)
Multivitamin
Digestive enzymes

Meal 2: Midmorning snack
(about 250 calories)
1 handful blueberries, 1 handful almonds, 1 handful beef jerky

Meal 3: Sun-Dried Tomato Chicken
(about 400 calories)
Add ½ cup steamed red peppers and ½ cup steamed broccoli on the side.
Digestive enzymes

Meal 4: Midafternoon snack
(about 200 calories)
1 apple, 1 low-sugar, high-fiber protein bar (preferably with a ratio of 1g fiber/1g protein, but no less than .5g/1g)

Meal 5: Spinach Egg-White Omelet
(about 400 calories)
Digestive enzymes

Meal 6: Pre/Postworkout snack
(about 250 calories)
1 banana with 1 tablespoon peanut butter and ¼ protein shake (1 scoop vanilla whey protein with water only) 45 to 30 minutes before workout, and the other ¾ protein shake after workout

Day 20 Friday

Drink 16 ounces water.

Meal 1: Spinach Shake
(about 400 calories)
Multivitamin
Digestive enzymes

Meal 2: Midmorning snack
(about 200 calories)
1 large handful almonds,
1 handful strawberries,

Meal 3: Sun-Dried Tomato Chicken on a salad (about 450 calories)
Place ½ cup leftover Sun-Dried Tomato Chicken, 1 small handful cashews, 1 handful blueberries, and 1 handful strawberries on a mixed dark green salad with a low-calorie vinaigrette dressing. (Raspberry vinaigrette goes well with berry salads.)
Digestive enzymes

Meal 4: Midafternoon snack
(about 300 calories)
1 grapefruit, 1 handful roasted pecans, 1 handful beef jerky

Meal 5: Citrus Salmon with Avocado Salsa (about 450 calories)
Add 1 cup steamed yellow squash on the side.
Digestive enzymes

Meal 6: Pre/Postworkout snack
(about 300 calories)
1 slice whole-wheat toast with 1 tablespoon peanut butter and ¼ protein shake (1 scoop vanilla whey protein with water only) 45 to 30 minutes before workout, and the other ¾ protein shake after workout

Day 21 Saturday

Drink 16 ounces water.

Meal 1: Farmer's Breakfast Scramble (about 550 calories)
Multivitamin
Digestive enzymes

Meal 2: Midmorning snack (about 250 calories)
1 large handful almonds, 1 handful beef jerky, 1 handful blueberries

Meal 3: Citrus Salmon with Avocado Salsa on a salad (about 450 calories)
Place 1 leftover fillet of Citrus Salmon on a mixed dark green salad with leftover Avocado Salsa.
Digestive enzymes

Meal 4: Midafternoon snack (about 350 calories)
1 banana with 2 tablespoons natural peanut butter, 1 small handful pumpkin seeds

Meal 5: ★Cheat/Treat Meal★ (about 700 calories)
Eat whatever you want as long as your other four meals today were nutritious, but try to keep it under 700 calories.
Digestive enzymes

Day 22 Sunday

Drink 16 ounces water.

Meal 1: Farmer's Breakfast Scramble (about 550 calories)
Multivitamin
Digestive enzymes

Meal 2: Midmorning snack (about 300 calories)
1 handful blueberries, 1 handful almonds, 1 low-sugar, high-fiber protein bar (preferably with a ratio of 1g fiber/1g protein, but no less than .5g/1g)

Meal 3: Spinach Shake (about 400 calories)
Digestive enzymes

Meal 4: Midafternoon snack (about 250 calories)
Celery with 2 tablespoons natural peanut butter, 1 handful raspberries

Meal 5: Basil Chicken with Vegetables (about 450 calories)*
Digestive enzymes

---

* Make enough of this recipe to last for three meals and refrigerate leftovers in tightly sealed containers for use later in the week.

Day 23 Monday

Drink 16 ounces water.

Meal 1: Pumpkin Pie Protein Shake (about 300 calories)
Multivitamin
Digestive enzymes

Meal 2: Midmorning snack (about 400 calories)
1 banana with 2 tablespoons natural peanut butter, 1 low-sugar, high-fiber protein bar (preferably with a ratio of 1g fiber/1g protein, but no less than .5g/1g)

Meal 3: Basil Chicken with Vegetables (about 450 calories)
Digestive enzymes

Meal 4: Midafternoon snack (about 200 calories)
1 grapefruit, 1 handful cashews

Meal 5: Sea Salt Salmon with Olive Oil Mayo (about 450 calories)
Add 1 cup steamed cauliflower on the side.
Digestive enzymes

Meal 6: Pre/Postworkout snack (about 300 calories)
1 slice whole-wheat toast with 1 tablespoon peanut butter and ¼ protein shake (1 scoop vanilla whey protein with water only) 45 to 30 minutes before workout, and the other ¾ protein shake after workout

Day 24 Tuesday

Drink 16 ounces water.

Meal 1: Spinach Shake (about 400 calories)
Multivitamin
Digestive enzymes

Meal 2: Midmorning snack (about 250 calories)
Celery with 2 tablespoons natural peanut butter, 1 apple

Meal 3: Basil Chicken with Vegetables on a salad (about 450 calories)
Place 1 cup leftover Basil Chicken with Vegetables over a mixed dark green salad with an oil-based vinaigrette dressing.
Digestive enzymes

Meal 4: Midafternoon snack (about 250 calories)
1 handful blueberries, 1 handful beef jerky, 1 handful pumpkin seeds

Meal 5: Spinach Egg-White Omelet (about 400 calories)
Digestive enzymes

Meal 6: Pre/Postworkout snack (about 250 calories)
1 banana with 1 tablespoon peanut butter and ¼ protein shake (1 scoop vanilla whey protein with water only) 45 to 30 minutes before workout, and the other ¾ protein shake after workout

Day 25 Wednesday

Drink 16 ounces water.

Meal 1: Spinach Shake
(about 400 calories)
Multivitamin
Digestive enzymes

Meal 2: Midmorning snack
(about 300 calories)
1 handful raspberries, 1 handful pumpkin seeds, 1 low-sugar, high-fiber protein bar (preferably with a ratio of 1g fiber/1g protein, but no less than .5g/1g)

Meal 3: Turkey Breast and Berry Salad (about 400 calories)
Digestive enzymes

Meal 4: Midafternoon snack
(about 250 calories)
1 banana with 2 tablespoons natural peanut butter

Meal 5: Beef Fajitas
(about 450 calories)*
Add 1 cup steamed yellow squash.
Digestive enzymes

Meal 6: Pre/Postworkout snack
(about 300 calories)
1 slice whole-wheat toast with 1 tablespoon peanut butter and ¼ protein shake (1 scoop vanilla whey protein with water only) 45 to 30 minutes before workout, and the other ¾ protein shake after workout

* Make enough of this recipe to last for three meals and refrigerate leftovers in tightly sealed containers for use later in the week.

Day 26 Thursday

Drink 16 ounces water.

Meal 1: Farmer's Breakfast Scramble
(about 550 calories)
Multivitamin
Digestive enzymes

Meal 2: Midmorning snack
(about 250 calories)
1 apple, 1 handful almonds, 1 handful beef jerky

Meal 3: Beef Fajitas
(about 450 calories)
Add 1 cup steamed yellow squash.
Digestive enzymes

Meal 4: Midafternoon snack
(about 300 calories)
1 handful pumpkin seeds, 1 handful blueberries, 1 low-sugar, high-fiber protein bar (preferably with a ratio of 1g fiber/1g protein, but no less than .5g/1g)

Meal 5: Spinach Shake
(about 400 calories)
Digestive enzymes

Meal 6: Pre/Postworkout snack
(about 250 calories)
1 banana with 1 tablespoon peanut butter and ¼ protein shake (1 scoop vanilla whey protein with water only) 45 to 30 minutes before workout, and the other ¾ protein shake after workout

Day 27 Friday

Drink 16 ounces water.

Meal 1: Spinach Shake
(about 400 calories)
Multivitamin
Digestive enzymes

Meal 2: Midmorning snack
(about 300 calories)
1 handful pumpkin seeds, 1 handful blueberries, 1 low-sugar, high-fiber protein bar (preferably with a ratio of 1g fiber/1g protein, but no less than .5g/1g)

Meal 3: Beef Fajitas on a salad
(about 400 calories)
Place 1 cup leftover Beef Fajitas meat and ¼ cup sliced red pepper (or a blend of red and yellow peppers) on a mixed dark green salad with an oil-based vinaigrette dressing.
Digestive enzymes

Meal 4: Midafternoon snack
(about 250 calories)
1 handful almonds, 1 handful beef jerky, 1 handful blueberries

Meal 5: Caramelized Onion–Glazed Salmon (about 450 calories)
Add 1 cup steamed zucchini on the side.
Digestive enzymes

Meal 6: Pre/Postworkout snack
(about 300 calories)
1 slice whole-wheat toast with 1 tablespoon peanut butter and ¼ protein shake (1 scoop vanilla whey protein with water only) 45 to 30 minutes before workout, and the other ¾ protein shake after workout

Day 28 Saturday

Drink 16 ounces water.

Meal 1: Farmer's Breakfast Scramble
(about 550 calories)
Multivitamin
Digestive enzymes

Meal 2: Midmorning snack
(about 250 calories)
1 grapefruit, 1 low-sugar, high-fiber protein bar (preferably with a ratio of 1g fiber/1g protein, but no less than .5g/1g)

Meal 3: Spinach Shake
(about 400 calories)
Digestive enzymes

Meal 4: Midafternoon snack
(about 350 calories)
1 apple with 2 tablespoons natural peanut butter, 1 handful pumpkin seeds

Meal 5: Caramelized Onion–Glazed Salmon (about 450 calories)
Place 1 fillet of leftover Caramelized Onion–Glazed Salmon on a mixed dark green salad with an oil-based vinaigrette dressing.
Digestive enzymes

Meal Plan 3: The Breakthrough

The following monthlong meal plan is designed specifically for when you've been progressing in your weight loss and total health journey, but seem to have hit a wall, even though you're doing everything right. This meal plan is not as balanced as the one you should use when you're maintaining—like in meal plan 2—but it's great for helping you push through to continue seeing results. I used a similar version of this for months 5 and 6, the conclusion of my journey from Fat2Fit. I still reintegrate this plan every few months to help me achieve my goals, or if I don't seem to be progressing.

Remember that I believe we should eat about every three hours throughout the day. Obviously, schedules for all of us are different, but the goal is to achieve a balanced regimen. Do your best to fit meals in on an every-three-hours rotation. Also, remember that you can mix and match (substitute) meals as you wish as long as the nutrition and calorie count stay the same.

As in the previous meal plans, women should reduce the overall daily caloric intake. In this particular plan, the reduction should be about 350 calories, accomplished by reducing portion size or by omitting some foods/snacks altogether.

You'll notice in this meal plan that the amount of protein increases in your pre- and postworkout meal. This is to ensure you're getting enough protein in before and after the workout, which will aid in muscle growth and recovery. Also, since this is a very low-carb meal plan, the added scoop of protein will add some needed calories for this sixth meal. You may also notice there are no built-in cheat/treat meals this month. Again, this is to push through the wall: no sacrifice, no reward!

Day 1 Sunday*

The first thing to do upon waking up is to drink 16 ounces of water. As with all of my meal plans, I focus on hydration right away in the morning.

Meal 1: Spinach Egg-White Omelet (about 400 calories)
Multivitamin
Digestive enzymes

Meal 2: Midmorning snack (about 200 calories)
1 handful blueberries,
1 large handful almonds

Meal 3: Pumpkin Pie Protein Shake (about 300 calories)
Digestive enzymes

Meal 4: Midafternoon snack (about 300 calories)
Celery with 2 tablespoons natural peanut butter, 1 handful roasted pecans

Meal 5: Thai Turkey Skillet (about 500 calories)**
Digestive enzymes

* Though we start the meal plan on Sunday, you can of course start any day of the week. The meal plan is outlined to cook a bulk of your meats in advance on Sunday and then again midweek on Wednesday. Feel free to adjust as needed.

** Make enough of this recipe to last for three meals and refrigerate leftovers in tightly sealed containers for use later in the week.

Day 2 Monday

Drink 16 ounces water.

Meal 1: Spinach Shake without the ½ banana (about 375 calories)
Multivitamin
Digestive enzymes

Meal 2: Midmorning snack (about 200 calories)
1 handful raspberries,
1 large handful almonds

Meal 3: Thai Turkey Skillet (about 500 calories)
Digestive enzymes

Meal 4: Midafternoon snack (about 250 calories)
1 large handful pumpkin seeds,
1 handful beef jerky

Meal 5: Caramelized Onion–Glazed Salmon (about 450 calories)
Add 2 cups steamed zucchini on the side.
Digestive enzymes

Meal 6: Pre/Postworkout snack (about 250 calories)
½ protein shake (2 scoops vanilla whey protein with water only) 45 to 30 minutes before workout, and the other ½ protein shake after workout. Also, include another multivitamin postworkout.

Day 3 Tuesday

Drink 16 ounces water.

Meal 1: Egg-White Breakfast Burrito without the tortilla (about 450 calories)
Multivitamin
Digestive enzymes

Meal 2: Midmorning snack (about 200 calories)
1 handful strawberries,
1 large handful almonds

Meal 3: Thai Turkey Skillet (about 500 calories)
Digestive enzymes

Meal 4: Midafternoon snack (about 200 calories)
3 rolled slices turkey lunch meat dipped in mustard, 1 handful almonds

Meal 5: Spinach Shake without the ½ banana (about 375 calories)
Digestive enzymes

Meal 6: Pre/Postworkout snack (about 250 calories)
½ protein shake (2 scoops vanilla whey protein with water only) 45 to 30 minutes before workout, and the other ½ protein shake after workout. Also, include another multivitamin postworkout.

---

* Make enough of this recipe to last for three meals and refrigerate leftovers in tightly sealed containers for use later in the week.

Day 4 Wednesday

Drink 16 ounces water.

Meal 1: Spinach Shake without the ½ banana (about 375 calories)
Multivitamin
Digestive enzymes

Meal 2: Midmorning snack (about 300 calories)
1 handful strawberries, 1 handful pumpkin seeds, 1 low-sugar, high-fiber protein bar (preferably with a ratio of 1g fiber/1g protein, but no less than .5g/1g)

Meal 3: Turkey Breast and Berry Salad (about 400 calories)
Digestive enzymes

Meal 4: Midafternoon snack (about 300 calories)
Celery with 2 tablespoons natural peanut butter, 1 handful roasted pecans

Meal 5: Sun-Dried Tomato Chicken (about 400 calories)*
Add 2 cups steamed asparagus on the side.
Digestive enzymes

Meal 6: Pre/Postworkout snack (about 250 calories)
½ protein shake (2 scoops vanilla whey protein with water only) 45 to 30 minutes before workout, and the other ½ protein shake after workout. Also, include another multivitamin postworkout.

Day 5 Thursday

Drink 16 ounces water.

Meal 1: Spinach Egg-White Omelet (about 400 calories)
Multivitamin
Digestive enzymes

Meal 2: Midmorning snack (about 200 calories)
1 handful strawberries,
1 large handful beef jerky

Meal 3: Sun-Dried Tomato Chicken (about 400 calories)
Add 2 cups steamed broccoli on the side.
Digestive enzymes

Meal 4: Midafternoon snack (about 250 calories)
3 rolled slices turkey lunch meat dipped in mustard, 1 large handful cashews

Meal 5: Turkey Breast and Berry Salad (about 400 calories)
Digestive enzymes

Meal 6: Pre/Postworkout snack (about 250 calories)
½ protein shake (2 scoops vanilla whey protein with water only) 45 to 30 minutes before workout, and the other ½ protein shake after workout. Also, include another multivitamin postworkout.

Day 6 Friday

Drink 16 ounces water.

Meal 1: Spinach Shake without the ½ banana (about 375 calories)
Multivitamin
Digestive enzymes

Meal 2: Midmorning snack (about 200 calories)
1 handful blueberries, 1 low-sugar, high-fiber protein bar (preferably with a ratio of 1g fiber/1g protein, but no less than .5g/1g)

Meal 3: Sun-Dried Tomato Chicken on a salad (about 450 calories)
Place 1 cup leftover Sun-Dried Tomato Chicken with ¼ cup chopped red pepper on a mixed dark green salad with an oil-based vinaigrette dressing.
Digestive enzymes

Meal 4: Midafternoon snack (about 300 calories)
1 handful almonds, celery with 2 tablespoons natural peanut butter

Meal 5: Citrus Salmon with Avocado Salsa (about 450 calories)
Add 2 cups steamed broccoli on the side.
Digestive enzymes

Meal 6: Pre/Postworkout snack (about 250 calories)
½ protein shake (2 scoops vanilla whey protein with water only) 45 to 30 minutes before workout, and the other ½ protein shake after workout. Also, include another multivitamin postworkout.

Day 7 Saturday

Drink 16 ounces water.

Meal 1: Pumpkin Pie Protein Shake
(about 300 calories)
Multivitamin
Digestive enzymes

Meal 2: Midmorning snack
(about 250 calories)
1 large handful almonds,
1 handful beef jerky

Meal 3: Spinach Egg-White Omelet
(about 400 calories)
Digestive enzymes

Meal 4: Midafternoon snack
(about 200 calories)
3 rolled slices turkey lunch meat dipped in mustard, 1 handful pumpkin seeds

Meal 5: Spinach Shake without the ½ banana (about 375 calories)
Digestive enzymes

Day 8 Sunday

Drink 16 ounces water.

Meal 1: Pumpkin Pie Protein Shake
(about 300 calories)
Multivitamin
Digestive enzymes

Meal 2: Midmorning snack
(about 250 calories)
1 handful pumpkin seeds, 1 low-sugar, high-fiber protein bar (preferably with a ratio of 1g fiber/1g protein, but no less than .5g/1g)

Meal 3: Spinach Egg-White Omelet
(about 400 calories)
Digestive enzymes

Meal 4: Midafternoon snack
(about 250 calories)
1 handful blueberries, 1 handful almonds, 1 handful beef jerky

Meal 5: Cajun Chicken Stir-Fry
(about 450 calories)*
Add 2 cups steamed cauliflower on the side.
Digestive enzymes

---

* Make enough of this recipe to last for three meals and refrigerate leftovers in tightly sealed containers for use later in the week.

Day 9 Monday

Drink 16 ounces water.

Meal 1: Spinach Shake without the ½ banana (about 375 calories)
Multivitamin
Digestive enzymes

Meal 2: Midmorning snack (about 350 calories)
Celery with 2 tablespoons natural peanut butter, 1 large handful almonds

Meal 3: Cajun Chicken Stir-Fry on a salad (about 450 calories)
Place about 1 cup leftover Cajun Chicken and ¼ cup chopped red peppers on a mixed dark green salad with an oil-based vinaigrette dressing.
Digestive enzymes

Meal 4: Midafternoon snack (about 250 calories)
3 rolled slices turkey lunch meat dipped in mustard, 1 large handful pumpkin seeds

Meal 5: Sea Salt Salmon with Olive Oil Mayo (about 450 calories)
Add 2 cups steamed asparagus on the side.
Digestive enzymes

Meal 6: Pre/Postworkout snack (about 250 calories)
½ protein shake (2 scoops vanilla whey protein with water only) 45 to 30 minutes before workout, and the other ½ protein shake after workout. Also, include another multivitamin postworkout.

Day 10 Tuesday

Drink 16 ounces water.

Meal 1: Egg-White Breakfast Burrito without the tortilla (about 450 calories)
Multivitamin
Digestive enzymes

Meal 2: Midmorning snack (about 250 calories)
1 grapefruit, 1 low-sugar, high-fiber protein bar (preferably with a ratio of 1g fiber/1g protein, but no less than .5g/1g)

Meal 3: Cajun Chicken Stir-Fry (about 450 calories)
Add 2 cups steamed asparagus on the side.
Digestive enzymes

Meal 4: Midafternoon snack (about 200 calories)
1 handful beef jerky,
1 handful pumpkin seeds

Meal 5: Spinach Shake without the ½ banana (about 375 calories)
Digestive enzymes

Meal 6: Pre/Postworkout snack (about 250 calories)
½ protein shake (2 scoops vanilla whey protein with water only) 45 to 30 minutes before workout, and the other ½ protein shake after workout. Also, include another multivitamin postworkout.

Day 11 Wednesday

Drink 16 ounces water.

Meal 1: Spinach Shake without the ½ banana (about 375 calories)
Multivitamin
Digestive enzymes

Meal 2: Midmorning snack (about 200 calories)
1 handful blueberries,
1 large handful roasted pecans

Meal 3: Turkey Breast and Berry Salad (about 400 calories)
Digestive enzymes

Meal 4: Midafternoon snack (about 250 calories)
3 rolled slices turkey lunch meat dipped in mustard, 1 large handful pumpkin seeds

Meal 5: Beef Fajitas (about 450 calories)*
Add 2 cups steamed yellow squash.
Digestive enzymes

Meal 6: Pre/Postworkout snack (about 250 calories)
½ protein shake (2 scoops vanilla whey protein with water only) 45 to 30 minutes before workout, and the other ½ protein shake after workout. Also, include another multivitamin postworkout.

---

* Make enough of this recipe to last for three meals and refrigerate leftovers in tightly sealed containers for use later in the week.

Day 12 Thursday

Drink 16 ounces water.

Meal 1: Spinach Shake without the ½ banana (about 375 calories)
Multivitamin
Digestive enzymes

Meal 2: Midmorning snack (about 300 calories)
1 handful almonds, 1 handful strawberries, 1 low-sugar, high-fiber protein bar (preferably with a ratio of 1g fiber/1g protein, but no less than .5g/1g)

Meal 3: Beef Fajitas (about 450 calories)
Add 2 cups steamed green beans on the side.
Digestive enzymes

Meal 4: Midafternoon snack (about 300 calories)
Celery with 2 tablespoons natural peanut butter, 1 handful cashews

Meal 5: Spinach Egg-White Omelet (about 400 calories)
Digestive enzymes

Meal 6: Pre/Postworkout snack (about 250 calories)
½ protein shake (2 scoops vanilla whey protein with water only) 45 to 30 minutes before workout, and the other ½ protein shake after workout. Also, include another multivitamin postworkout.

Day 13 Friday

Drink 16 ounces water.

Meal 1: Spinach Shake without the ½ banana (about 375 calories)
Multivitamin
Digestive enzymes

Meal 2: Midmorning snack (about 300 calories)
1 handful almonds, 1 handful strawberries, 1 low-sugar, high-fiber protein bar (preferably with a ratio of 1g fiber/1g protein, but no less than .5g/1g)

Meal 3: Beef Fajitas on a salad (about 500 calories)
Place 1 cup leftover Beef Fajitas meat, ¼ cup sliced pepper (your choice), and ¼ cup sliced avocado on a mixed dark green salad with an oil-based vinaigrette dressing.
Digestive enzymes

Meal 4: Midafternoon snack (about 300 calories)
1 handful pumpkin seeds,
Celery with 2 tablespoons natural peanut butter

Meal 5: Caramelized Onion–Glazed Salmon (about 450 calories)
Add 2 cups steamed broccoli on the side.
Digestive enzymes

Meal 6: Pre/Postworkout snack (about 250 calories)
½ protein shake (2 scoops vanilla whey protein with water only) 45 to 30 minutes before workout, and the other ½ protein shake after workout. Also, include another multivitamin postworkout.

Day 14 Saturday

Drink 16 ounces water.

Meal 1: Pumpkin Pie Protein Shake
(about 300 calories)
Multivitamin
Digestive enzymes

Meal 2: Midmorning snack
(about 250 calories)
1 handful almonds, 1 handful beef jerky, 1 handful blueberries

Meal 3: Spinach Egg-White Omelet
(about 400 calories)
Digestive enzymes

Meal 4: Midafternoon snack
(about 200 calories)
3 rolled slices turkey lunch meat dipped in mustard, 1 handful pumpkin seeds

Meal 5: Caramelized Onion–Glazed Salmon on a salad (about 500 calories)
Serve 1 fillet of leftover Caramelized Onion–Glazed Salmon over a mixed dark green salad with an oil-based vinaigrette dressing.
Digestive enzymes

Day 15 Sunday

Drink 16 ounces water.

Meal 1: Pumpkin Pie Protein Shake
(about 300 calories)
Multivitamin
Digestive enzymes

Meal 2: Midmorning snack
(about 250 calories)
1 handful pumpkin seeds, 1 low-sugar, high-fiber protein bar (preferably with a ratio of 1g fiber/1g protein, but no less than .5g/1g)

Meal 3: Egg-White Breakfast Burrito without the tortilla (about 500 calories)
Digestive enzymes

Meal 4: Midafternoon snack
(about 200 calories)
1 handful almonds,
1 handful beef jerky

Meal 5: Mexican Chicken
(about 450 calories)*
Add 2 cups steamed cauliflower on the side.
Digestive enzymes

---

* Make enough of this recipe to last for three meals and refrigerate leftovers in tightly sealed containers for use later in the week.

Day 16 Monday

Drink 16 ounces water.

Meal 1: Spinach Shake without the ½ banana (about 375 calories)
Multivitamin
Digestive enzymes

Meal 2: Midmorning snack (about 200 calories)
1 handful raspberries,
1 large handful almonds

Meal 3: Mexican Chicken (about 450 calories)
Add 2 cups steamed cauliflower on the side.
Digestive enzymes

Meal 4: Midafternoon snack (about 200 calories)
3 rolled slices turkey lunch meat dipped in mustard, 1 handful pumpkin seeds

Meal 5: Sea Salt Salmon with Olive Oil Mayo (about 450 calories)
Add 2 cups steamed asparagus on the side.
Digestive enzymes

Meal 6: Pre/Postworkout snack (about 250 calories)
½ protein shake (2 scoops vanilla whey protein with water only) 45 to 30 minutes before workout, and the other ½ protein shake after workout. Also, include another multivitamin postworkout.

Day 17 Tuesday

Drink 16 ounces water.

Meal 1: Egg-White Breakfast Burrito without the tortilla (about 450 calories)
Multivitamin
Digestive enzymes

Meal 2: Midmorning snack (about 250 calories)
1 handful blueberries, 1 handful roasted pecans, 1 handful beef jerky

Meal 3: Mexican Chicken on a salad (about 450 calories)
Place 1 cup leftover Mexican Chicken, ¼ cup sliced avocado, and ¼ cup sliced yellow pepper on a mixed dark green salad with an oil-based vinaigrette dressing.
Digestive enzymes

Meal 4: Midafternoon snack (about 250 calories)
1 handful almonds, 1 low-sugar, high-fiber protein bar (preferably with a ratio of 1g fiber/1g protein, but no less than .5g/1g)

Meal 5: Spinach Shake without the ½ banana (about 375 calories)
Digestive enzymes

Meal 6: Pre/Postworkout snack (about 250 calories)
½ protein shake (2 scoops vanilla whey protein with water only) 45 to 30 minutes before workout, and the other ½ protein shake after workout. Also, include another multivitamin postworkout.

Day 18 Wednesday

Drink 16 ounces water.

Meal 1: Spinach Shake without the ½ banana (about 375 calories)
Multivitamin
Digestive enzymes

Meal 2: Midmorning snack (about 200 calories)
1 handful blueberries,
1 large handful almonds

Meal 3: Turkey Breast and Berry Salad (about 400 calories)
Digestive enzymes

Meal 4: Midafternoon snack (about 200 calories)
3 rolled slices turkey lunch meat dipped in mustard, 1 handful roasted pecans

Meal 5: Sun-Dried Tomato Chicken (about 400 calories)*
Add 2 cups steamed green beans on the side.
Digestive enzymes

Meal 6: Pre/Postworkout snack (about 250 calories)
½ protein shake (2 scoops vanilla whey protein with water only) 45 to 30 minutes before workout, and the other ½ protein shake after workout. Also, include another multivitamin postworkout.

Day 19 Thursday

Drink 16 ounces water.

Meal 1: Spinach Shake without the ½ banana (about 375 calories)
Multivitamin
Digestive enzymes

Meal 2: Midmorning snack (about 250 calories)
1 handful blueberries, 1 handful almonds, 1 handful beef jerky

Meal 3: Sun-Dried Tomato Chicken (about 400 calories)
Add 1 cup steamed red peppers and 1 cup steamed broccoli on the side.
Digestive enzymes

Meal 4: Midafternoon snack (about 150 calories)
1 low-sugar, high-fiber protein bar (preferably with a ratio of 1g fiber/1g protein, but no less than .5g/1g)

Meal 5: Spinach Egg-White Omelet (about 400 calories)
Digestive enzymes

Meal 6: Pre/Postworkout snack (about 250 calories)
½ protein shake (2 scoops vanilla whey protein with water only) 45 to 30 minutes before workout, and the other ½ protein shake after workout. Also, include another multivitamin postworkout.

---

* Make enough of this recipe to last for three meals and refrigerate leftovers in tightly sealed containers for use later in the week.

Day 20 Friday

Drink 16 ounces water.

Meal 1: Spinach Shake without the ½ banana (about 375 calories)
Multivitamin
Digestive enzymes

Meal 2: Midmorning snack (about 250 calories)
1 large handful almonds, 3 rolled slices turkey lunch meat dipped in mustard

Meal 3: Sun-Dried Tomato Chicken on a salad (about 450 calories)
Place ½ cup leftover Sun-Dried Tomato Chicken, 1 small handful cashews, 1 handful blueberries, and 1 handful strawberries on a mixed dark green salad with low-calorie vinaigrette dressing. (Raspberry vinaigrette goes well with berry salads.)
Digestive enzymes

Meal 4: Midafternoon snack (about 200 calories)
1 handful roasted pecans,
1 handful beef jerky

Meal 5: Citrus Salmon with Avocado Salsa (about 450 calories)
Add 2 cups steamed broccoli on the side.
Digestive enzymes

Meal 6: Pre/Postworkout snack (about 250 calories)
½ protein shake (2 scoops vanilla whey protein with water only) 45 to 30 minutes before workout, and the other ½ protein shake after workout. Also, include another multivitamin postworkout.

Day 21 Saturday

Drink 16 ounces water.

Meal 1: Egg-White Breakfast Burrito without the tortilla (about 450 calories)
Multivitamin
Digestive enzymes

Meal 2: Midmorning snack (about 300 calories)
Celery with 2 tablespoons natural peanut butter, 1 handful beef jerky

Meal 3: Citrus Salmon with Avocado Salsa on a salad (about 450 calories)
Place 1 leftover fillet of Citrus Salmon on a mixed dark green salad with leftover Avocado Salsa.
Digestive enzymes

Meal 4: Midafternoon snack (about 250 calories)
3 rolled slices turkey lunch meat dipped in mustard, 1 large handful pumpkin seeds

Meal 5: Spinach Shake without the ½ banana (about 375 calories)
Digestive enzymes

Day 22 Sunday

Drink 16 ounces water.

Meal 1: Spinach Egg-White Omelet (about 400 calories)
Multivitamin
Digestive enzymes

Meal 2: Midmorning snack (about 300 calories)
1 handful blueberries, 1 handful almonds, 1 low-sugar, high-fiber protein bar (preferably with a ratio of 1g fiber/1g protein, but no less than .5g/1g)

Meal 3: Pumpkin Pie Protein Shake (about 300 calories)
Digestive enzymes

Meal 4: Midafternoon snack (about 300 calories)
Celery with 2 tablespoons natural peanut butter, 1 handful beef jerky

Meal 5: Chinese "Fried Rice" (about 450 calories)*
Digestive enzymes

---

* Make enough of this recipe to last for three meals and refrigerate leftovers in tightly sealed containers for use later in the week.

Day 23 Monday

Drink 16 ounces water.

Meal 1: Spinach Shake without the ½ banana (about 375 calories)
Multivitamin
Digestive enzymes

Meal 2: Midmorning snack (about 250 calories)
3 rolled slices turkey lunch meat dipped in mustard, 1 low-sugar, high-fiber protein bar (preferably with a ratio of 1g fiber/1g protein, but no less than .5g/1g)

Meal 3: Chinese "Fried Rice" (about 450 calories)
Digestive enzymes

Meal 4: Midafternoon snack (about 200 calories)
1 handful cashews,
1 handful beef jerky

Meal 5: Sea Salt Salmon with Olive Oil Mayo (about 450 calories)
Add 2 cups steamed green beans on the side.
Digestive enzymes

Meal 6: Pre/Postworkout snack (about 250 calories)
½ protein shake (2 scoops vanilla whey protein with water only) 45 to 30 minutes before workout, and the other ½ protein shake after workout. Also, include another multivitamin postworkout.

Day 24 Tuesday

Drink 16 ounces water.

Meal 1: Spinach Shake without the ½ banana (about 375 calories)
Multivitamin
Digestive enzymes

Meal 2: Midmorning snack (about 300 calories)
Celery with 2 tablespoons natural peanut butter, 3 rolled slices turkey lunch meat dipped in mustard

Meal 3: Chinese "Fried Rice" (about 450 calories)
Digestive enzymes

Meal 4: Midafternoon snack (about 250 calories)
1 handful beef jerky,
1 large handful pumpkin seeds

Meal 5: Spinach Egg-White Omelet (about 400 calories)
Digestive enzymes

Meal 6: Pre/Postworkout snack (about 250 calories)
½ protein shake (2 scoops vanilla whey protein with water only) 45 to 30 minutes before workout, and the other ½ protein shake after workout. Also, include another multivitamin postworkout.

Day 25 Wednesday

Drink 16 ounces water.

Meal 1: Spinach Shake without the ½ banana (about 375 calories)
Multivitamin
Digestive enzymes

Meal 2: Midmorning snack (about 200 calories)
1 handful pumpkin seeds, 1 handful almonds

Meal 3: Turkey Breast and Berry Salad (about 400 calories)
Digestive enzymes

Meal 4: Midafternoon snack (about 300 calories)
Celery with 2 tablespoons natural peanut butter, 1 handful beef jerky

Meal 5: Turkey Fajitas (substitute turkey breast for beef in the Beef Fajitas recipe) (about 450 calories)*
Add 2 cups steamed yellow squash.
Digestive enzymes

Meal 6: Pre/Postworkout snack (about 250 calories)
½ protein shake (2 scoops vanilla whey protein with water only) 45 to 30 minutes before workout, and the other ½ protein shake after workout. Also, include another multivitamin postworkout.

* Make enough of this recipe to last for three meals and refrigerate leftovers in tightly sealed containers for use later in the week.

Day 26 Thursday

Drink 16 ounces water.

Meal 1: Spinach Egg-White Omelet (about 400 calories)
Multivitamin
Digestive enzymes

Meal 2: Midmorning snack (about 250 calories)
1 large handful almonds, 1 handful beef jerky

Meal 3: Turkey Fajitas (about 450 calories)
Add 2 cups steamed yellow squash.
Digestive enzymes

Meal 4: Midafternoon snack (about 300 calories)
1 handful pumpkin seeds, 1 handful blueberries, 1 low-sugar, high-fiber protein bar (preferably with a ratio of 1g fiber/1g protein, but no less than .5g/1g)

Meal 5: Spinach Shake without the ½ banana (about 375 calories)
Digestive enzymes

Meal 6: Pre/Postworkout snack (about 250 calories)
½ protein shake (2 scoops vanilla whey protein with water only) 45 to 30 minutes before workout, and the other ½ protein shake after workout. Also, include another multivitamin postworkout.

Day 27 Friday

Drink 16 ounces water.

Meal 1: Spinach Shake without the ½ banana (about 375 calories)
Multivitamin
Digestive enzymes

Meal 2: Midmorning snack (about 200 calories)
3 rolled slices turkey lunch meat dipped in mustard, 1 handful pumpkin seeds

Meal 3: Turkey Fajitas on a salad (about 450 calories)
Place 1 cup leftover Turkey Fajitas meat and ¼ cup chopped red pepper (or a mix of red and yellow peppers) on a mixed dark green salad with an oil-based vinaigrette dressing.
Digestive enzymes

Meal 4: Midafternoon snack (about 250 calories)
1 large handful almonds,
1 handful beef jerky

Meal 5: Caramelized Onion–Glazed Salmon (about 450 calories)
Add 2 cups steamed zucchini on the side.
Digestive enzymes

Meal 6: Pre/Postworkout snack (about 250 calories)
½ protein shake (2 scoops vanilla whey protein with water only) 45 to 30 minutes before workout, and the other ½ protein shake after workout. Also, include another multivitamin postworkout.

Day 28 Saturday

Drink 16 ounces water.

Meal 1: Spinach Egg-White Omelet (about 400 calories)
Multivitamin
Digestive enzymes

Meal 2: Midmorning snack (about 300 calories)
Celery with 2 tablespoons natural peanut butter, 1 handful roasted pecans

Meal 3: Pumpkin Pie Protein Shake (about 300 calories)
Digestive enzymes

Meal 4: Midafternoon snack (about 250 calories)
3 rolled slices turkey lunch meat dipped in mustard, 1 large handful pumpkin seeds

Meal 5: Caramelized Onion–Glazed Salmon (about 450 calories)
Serve 1 fillet of leftover Caramelized Onion–Glazed Salmon on a mixed dark green salad with an oil-based vinaigrette dressing.
Digestive enzymes

EXERCISES

In this appendix I describe, in detail, some excellent exercises that are my personal favorites when it comes to getting fit. In the next section, titled "Workouts," I'll incorporate some of these exercises to provide detailed workouts, which will include the appropriate amount of repetitions ("reps") and sets. Look at the pictures as you read the instructions. The words and images together should help you master the motions.

Note that there is some overlap between these two appendices. Consult this one, "Exercises," if you're trying to get the basic motions down; consult "Workouts" once you've mastered these and are ready to put them together and begin working toward the new you.

Push-Ups with One Hand on Medicine Ball

I'm a big believer in keeping things simple. That's why push-ups will always be a staple in my exercises. I love feeling athletic, being able to do push-ups without feeling like I'm going to die after doing only 10! Push-ups on a medicine ball add a different dimension to boring old push-ups, and they allow you to get a deeper stretch in the pectoral muscles as well as strengthen the small stabilizer muscles in the shoulders. Adding a pulse at the bottom of the push-ups adds a degree of difficulty as well. Doing push-ups according to these instructions will definitely build strength, tone those chest muscles, and build endurance.

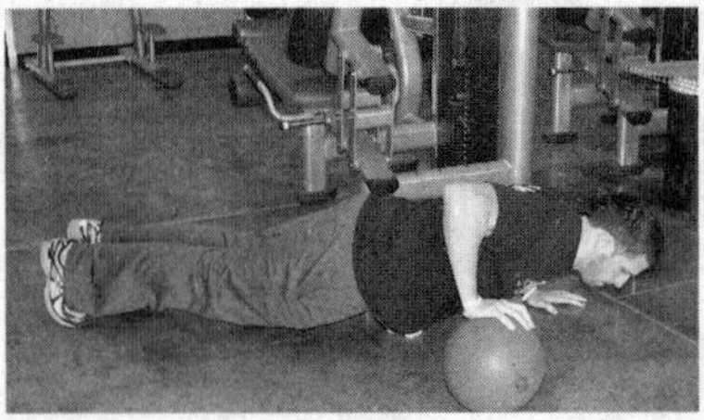

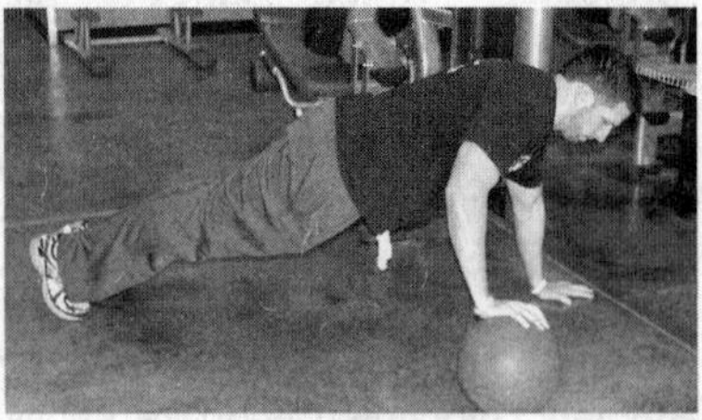

STEP 1 **With your body prone, place your hands on the floor so that they're about shoulder width apart, one hand on a medicine ball.**

STEP 2 **Rise up onto your toes so that all of your body weight is on your hands and feet.**

STEP 3 **Bring your body into a straight line and keep it that way throughout the exercise.**

STEP 4 **Bend your elbows and lower your chest toward the floor.**

STEP 5 **Once your elbows bend slightly beyond 90 degrees, push off the floor slightly and return immediately to the bottom again (a so-called pulse); then extend your arms all the way so that you return to the starting position.**

Dumbbell Bench Presses on Stability Ball (One Arm at a Time)

I like to focus on a lot of unilateral movements when it comes to my exercises. This helps with muscle imbalances, which are very common, and also helps to strengthen the small stabilizer muscles, which don't get worked out as often as the larger muscles. This exercise is another great chest workout; it allows you to isolate each chest muscle individually, and when you strengthen each component, you become stronger as a whole.

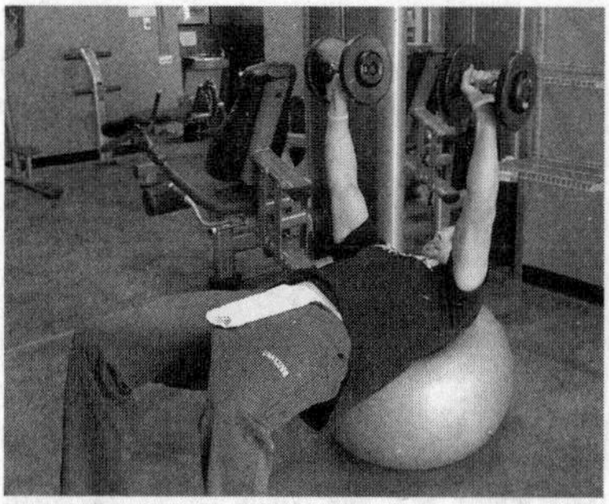

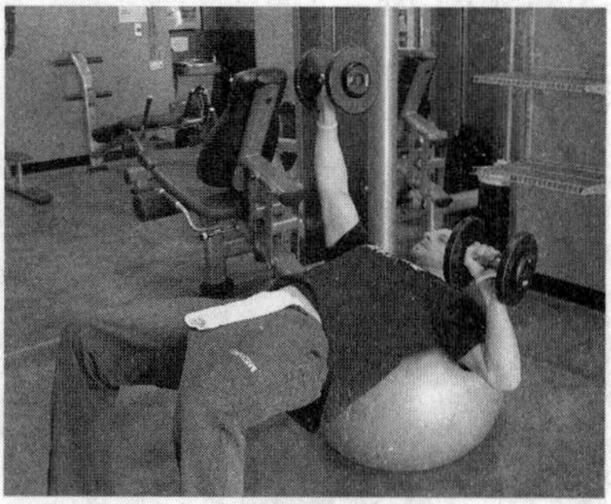

STEP 1 **Lie on your back on a medium- to large-size (55 to 75 cm) stability ball with knees bent so that your body is parallel to the floor. (Your upper back should be resting on the stability ball while your hips and butt will be off the medicine ball.)**

STEP 2 **With arms perpendicular to your body and bent upward at the elbow, hold the dumbbells out to the side.**

STEP 3 **Press both dumbbells up until arms are fully extended.**

STEP 4 **Lower one of the weights toward the side of your upper chest (keeping your other arm extended) until a slight stretch is felt in the chest or shoulder.**

STEP 5 **Finally, extend the arm fully to the step 3 position.
Now switch arms!**

Pull-Ups

Pull-ups are a must in my workout routine. Even if I'm trying to build more muscle mass, I still include this excellent exercise in whatever routine I'm doing. This is definitely a good measuring tool for me as far as my athleticism is concerned, and I'm always striving to be able to perform more repetitions of this exercise. Pull-ups work multiple muscles in the back, as well as the biceps, forearms, and even core. That's why this exercise is a must, especially for those who desire to achieve the upper-body V shape that many fitness buffs strive for.

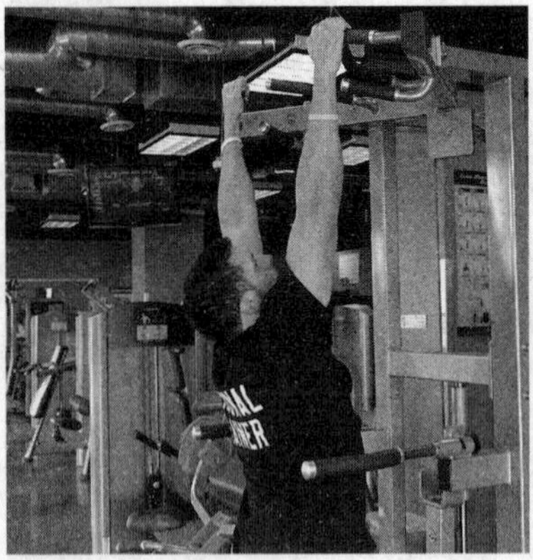

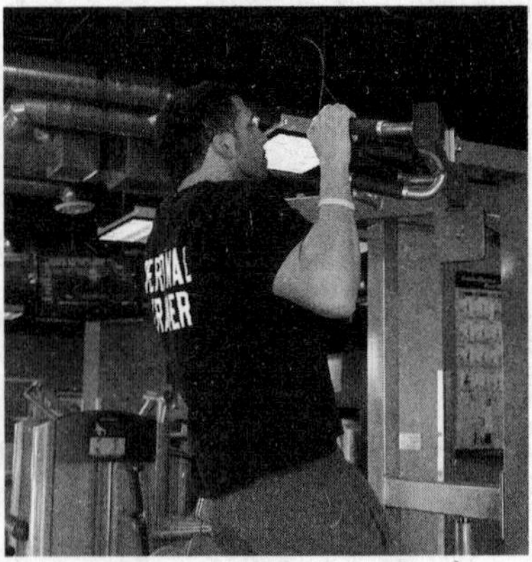

STEP 1 **Grip the pull-up bar with palms facing away from you.**

STEP 2 **Extend your arms all the way and hang from the bar.**

STEP 3 **Pull your body up (without a swinging motion) until your chin reaches above the bar.**

STEP 4 **Return to the starting position and repeat.**

Dumbbell Deadlifts

Deadlifts are an often-forgotten (or -neglected) exercise in the gym. I don't blame anyone for not wanting to perform these, because they're exhausting when done properly. However, dumbbell deadlifts are a great strengthening exercise for the lower back, middle back, upper back, core, legs, forearms, and grip strength. I generally perform these on those weight-training days that focus on my back.

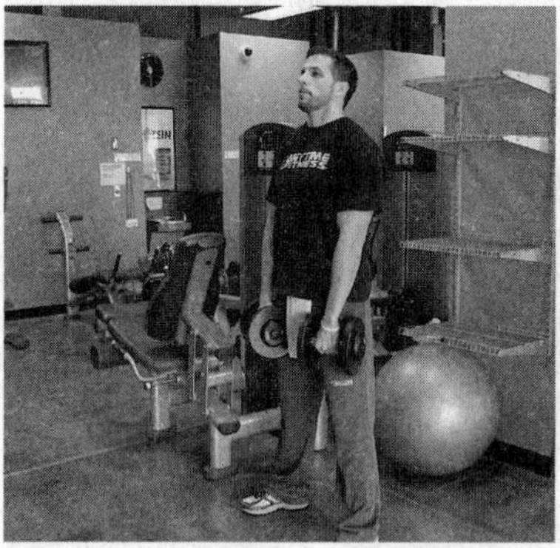

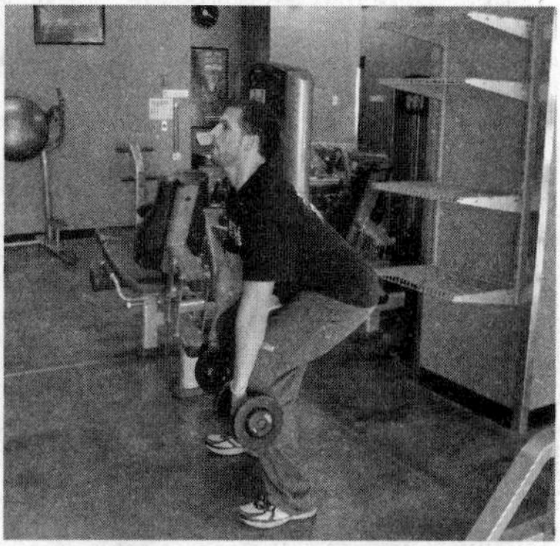

STEP 1 **Stand straight up, feet shoulder width apart, with dumbbells resting just in front of you, your arms fully extended downward.**

STEP 2 **Slowly lower the dumbbells while keeping your back straight (though angled forward), chest out, and butt back until the dumbbells go below the kneecaps.**

STEP 3 **Return to a fully standing position while keeping the dumbbells close to your body.**

Jumping Squats

Squats are another exercise that many people avoid, because their legs quickly feel like Jell-O after only the first set when squats are done properly. Like deadlifts, they benefit many muscle groups: lower back, quads, hamstrings, glutes, calves, and even abs. Some will argue that no other exercise works as many muscles as squats do. *Jumping* squats add a degree of difficulty, but in different ways than traditional barbell squats. This variation works the fast-twitch muscle fibers, and you won't want to be using nearly as much weight as in traditional squats. This is a great exercise you can do without a gym membership and without equipment. You'll be sweating and breathing hard after doing these no matter what your level of fitness!

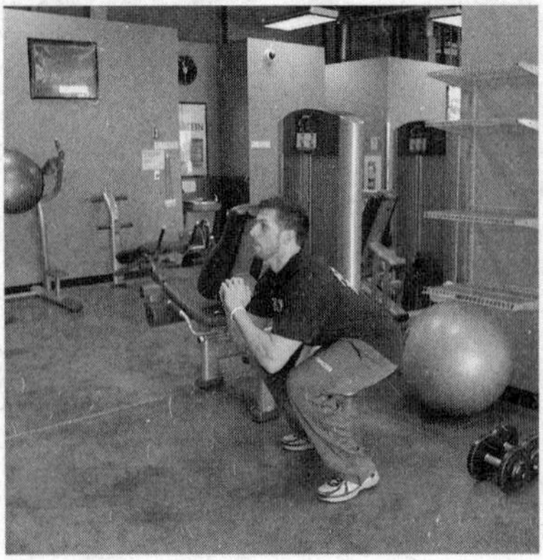

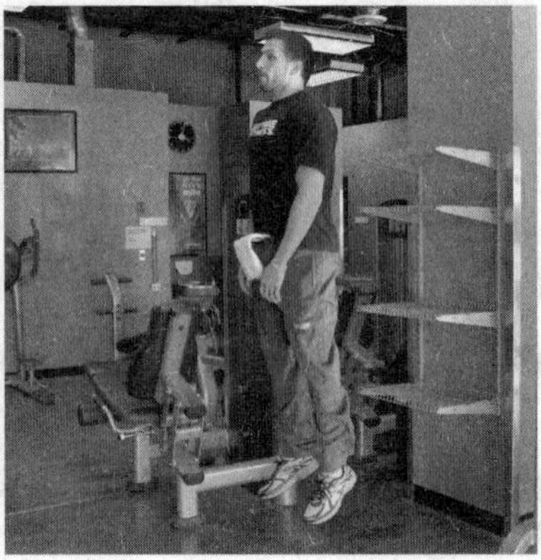

STEP 1 **Stand with feet shoulder width apart.**

STEP 2 **Lower your body while keeping your chest out, back straight, and butt back.**

STEP 3 **Go down until your thighs are parallel to the ground; then explode and jump up as high as you can.**

STEP 4 **Instead of landing with your legs locked straight, land with bent knees. Don't stop your motion, though; slowly lower yourself again and repeat the squat without pause (that is, no rest between).**

Jumping Lunges

Lunges are another great exercise to help strengthen the legs and glutes. Most men think lunges are for "girls," mostly because these exercises help to shape the glutes, but my opinion is that *no one* should have a saggy rear end. That's why leg days, for me, will always include some form of lunges. *Jumping* lunges, like jumping squats, add a slight degree of difficulty. They're very effective at burning calories during your workout and will definitely get your heart rate up, which is good for your cardiovascular system.

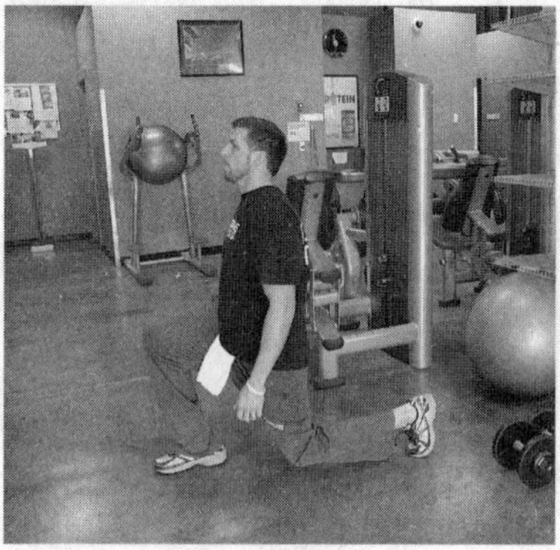

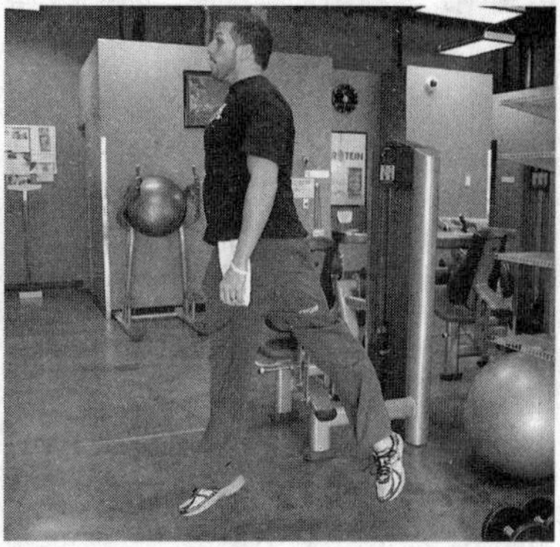

STEP 1 **Stand with one foot way out in front of you and the other back behind you, with the back foot up on your toes.**

STEP 2 **Go straight down, with back straight, until your front leg is parallel to the floor, making sure that your front knee doesn't go in front of your front toes.**

STEP 3 **From that lowest position, explode and jump up as high as you can.**

STEP 4 **Instead of landing with your legs locked straight, land with bent knees, switching legs each time you land (so that if your right leg was in back before the jump, it's now in front). Don't stop your motion, though; slowly lower yourself again and repeat without pausing.**

Side to Front to Side Dumbbell Raises

The title of this exercise might seem confusing, but it's actually two exercises—side dumbbell raises and front dumbbell raises—rolled into three simple motions. This is a solid endurance exercise as well as a great toning exercise for your side and front deltoids. I like to mix this one into my workouts to get a great burn.

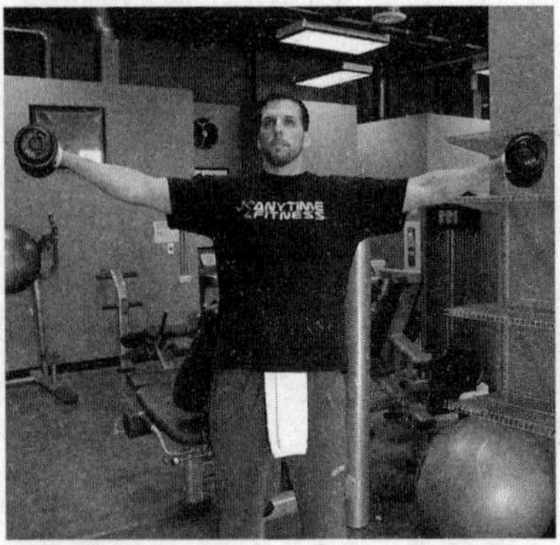

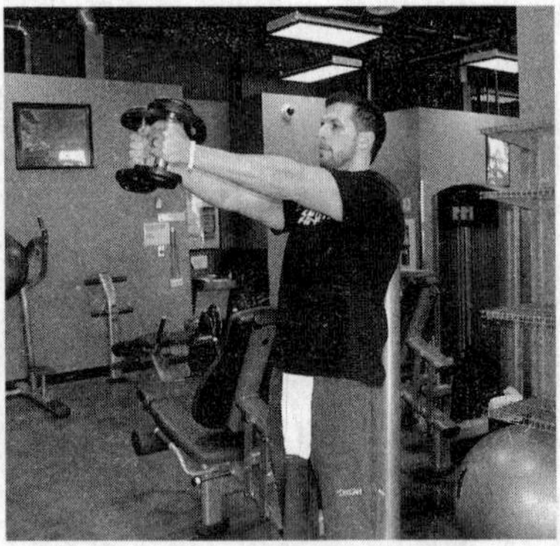

STEP 1 **Stand with feet shoulder width apart, with dumbbells hanging at your sides.**

STEP 2 **With elbows slightly bent raise both dumbbells to your sides, away from your body, until your arms are parallel to the floor.**

STEP 3 **Keeping your arms parallel to the floor, bring dumbbells in front of you until they touch (turning them so that they become perpendicular to the floor).**

STEP 4 **Still keeping arms parallel to the floor, bring dumbbells back out to the sides, and then lower down to your waist/hips.**

Hand Step-Ups with Plank

This is a great exercise that I was able to perform with Dr. Oz when I was on his show. It's another multimuscle exercise, but I tend to do it on my shoulder days. It covers a wide variety of muscles, including shoulders, triceps, and core, and it's also great for cardiovascular endurance. The word "plank" refers to the straight line your body maintains.

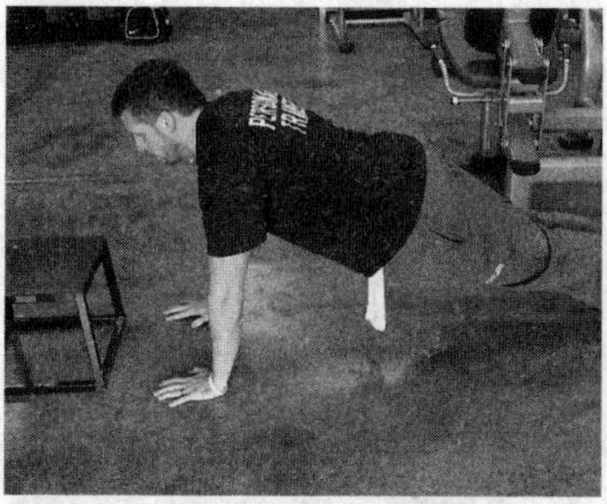

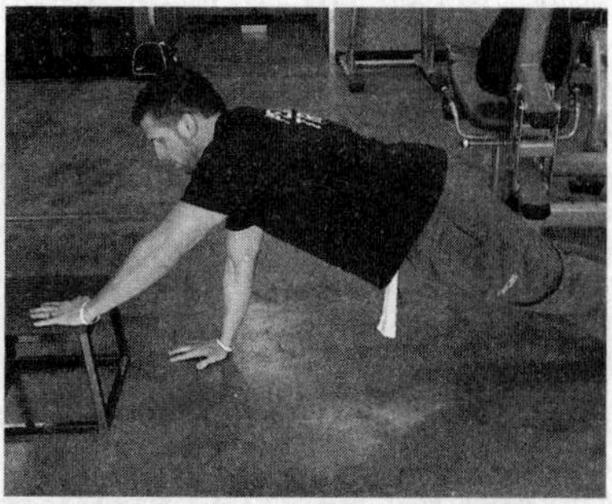

STEP 1 **Place a low step against a wall for stability, or use your stairs at home.**

STEP 2 **Now get in push-up position on the floor, facing the step in front of you. (If you're a beginner, you can do this exercise on your knees until you build up the strength to do it without the added assistance.)**

STEP 3 **Put one hand flat on the top of the step, followed by the other hand (keeping your body in a straight line—hence the word "plank").**

STEP 4 **Return hands down off the step/stair one at a time until you're back in the starting push-up position.**

STEP 5 **Repeat these movements at a fast pace for approximately 30 to 45 seconds, depending on your fitness level.**

Chin-Ups

This is another vital exercise to strengthen your upper body and improve your flexibility and athleticism. Chin-ups, which are different from pull-ups due to the way the palms are facing (pull-ups = palms facing away from you; chin-ups = palms facing toward you), allow you to focus more on the biceps muscles. This is why I always perform chin-ups on my biceps day instead of doing just a bunch of standard curls. This exercise strengthens so much more than just biceps, but it's a great way to get those "guns" for us men—or, for you ladies, it'll create some nice definition.

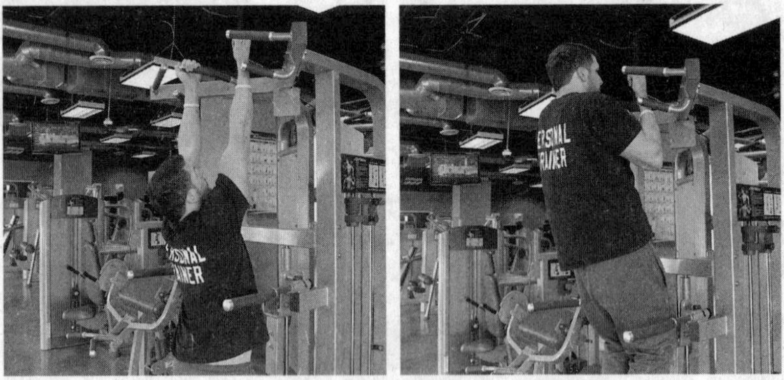

STEP 1 **Grip the pull-up bar with palms facing you.**

STEP 2 **Extend your arms all the way and hang from the bar.**

STEP 3 **Pull your body up (without a swinging motion), using primarily your biceps, until your chin reaches above the bar.**

STEP 4 **Return to the starting position and repeat.**

Dumbbell Curls

"Curls for the girls"—that's what my wrestling coach used to call these back in high school. Curls aren't that difficult to do, and they make your arms look defined. I like to add a few twists to traditional dumbbell curls, though. Adding a quick 1-count on the way up (positives) followed by a slow 3-count on the way down (negatives) is great for improved strength and explosiveness.

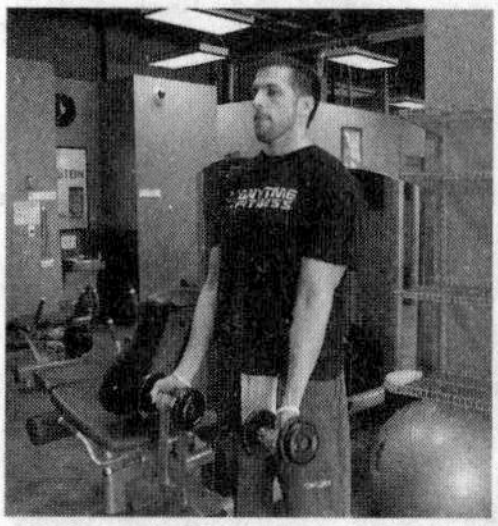
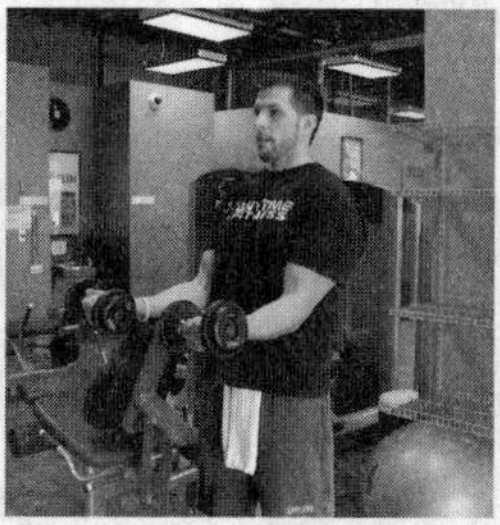
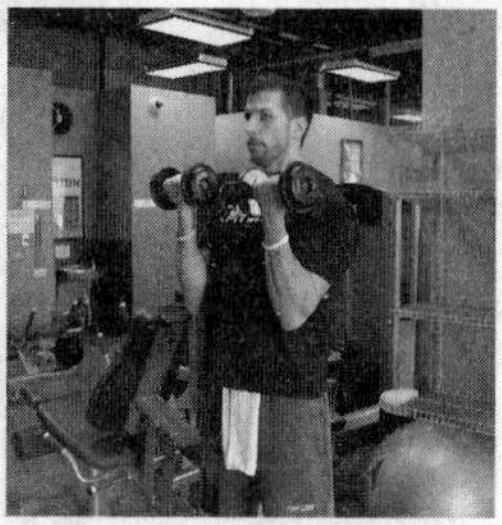

STEP 1 **Stand with feet shoulder width apart while holding dumbbells. Let the weights hang in front of you with your palms facing forward.**

STEP 2 **While keeping your back straight, bring dumbbells up in the curve of a D-shaped motion, using your biceps. At the top, squeeze/flex the biceps. (Do the lifting motion as you count to 1; it should be a fast motion.)**

STEP 3 **Return back down in the same D-shaped arc—this time counting to 3 to get a slow motion—until your arms are fully extended and back in the starting position.**

Dips with a Pulse

Dips are another great exercise I work into my routine no matter what phase I'm in (strength building vs. toning). There are many variations and degrees of difficulty for this exercise. I like to include a pulse at the bottom to add an extra degree of difficulty—and you'll feel better after even one set!

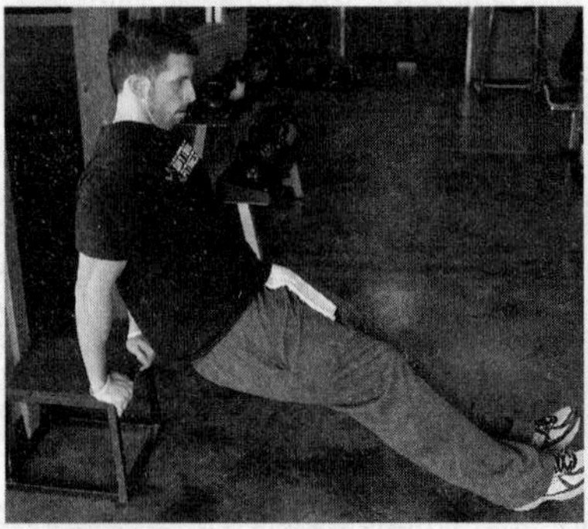

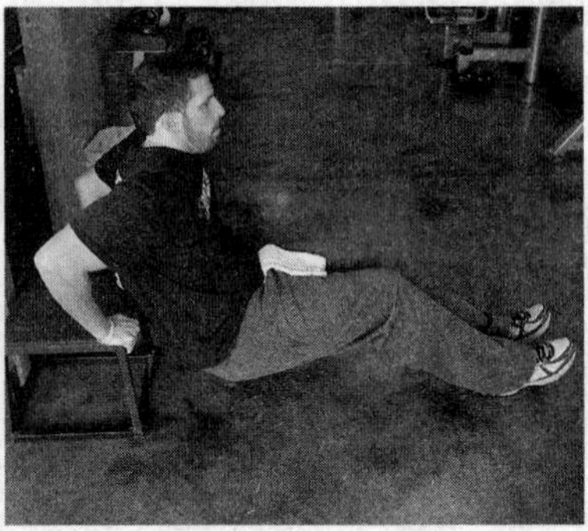

STEP 1 **Sit on a chair with your hands on the edges a bit out from your hips.**

STEP 2 **Walk your body away from the chair so that you're holding yourself up with your arms, and your feet are about shoulder width apart, giving you extra support.**

STEP 3 **Go straight down until your arms form a 90-degree angle (keeping your elbows in and your back straight).**

STEP 4 **Come back up slightly (about ¼ of the way), then return all the way back down again.**

STEP 5 **Return up to the starting position.**

Triceps "Skull Crushers"

Another great and effective triceps workout is "skull crushers," which sound intimidating but are pretty simple to do, even at home. This exercise really helps to isolate just the triceps muscles. Having stronger triceps will help with a lot of other upper-body exercises. My wife loves these; she says they help prevent those flabby arms that many women struggle with.

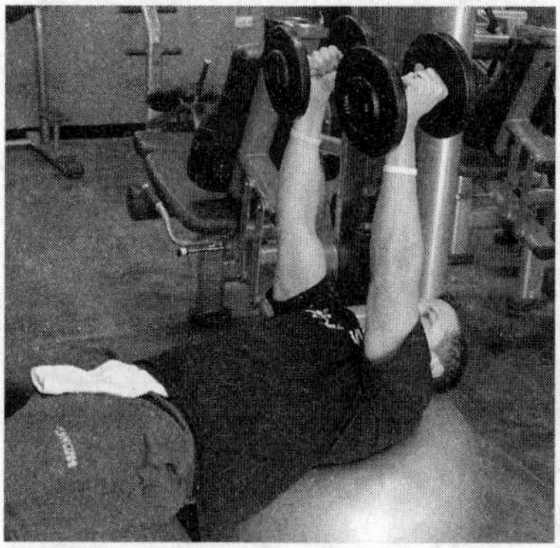

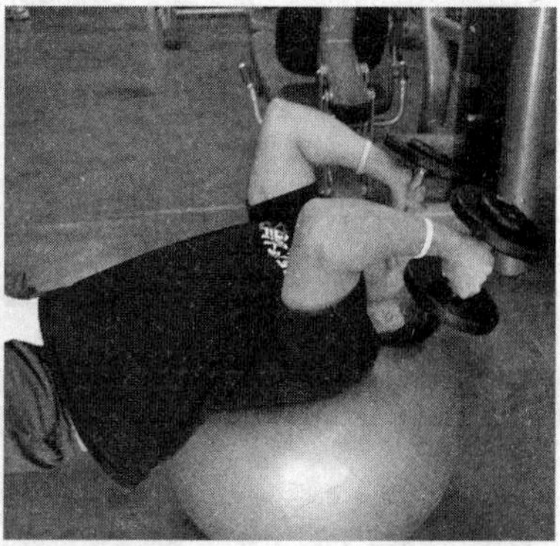

STEP 1 **Lie down with your back on a stability ball, knees bent as needed, so that your body is parallel to the floor.**

STEP 2 **Bring dumbbells straight up above your head with arms extended and palms facing each other.**

STEP 3 **Bend your arms to 90 degrees so that the dumbbells reach your forehead on both sides. (Don't actually hit your head; just get close!)**

STEP 4 **At the bottom do a pulse by bringing the dumbbells back up a quarter of the way, then back down all the way; then straighten your arms so that the dumbbells are again above you, keeping your elbows in the same position throughout the entire step.**

Planks with a Hip Rotation

Strengthening your core is one of the most important things when it comes to physical fitness, yet it's overlooked by many, including professional athletes. Your core is your foundation, and if *it* is strong, that strength will benefit the rest of your body. So many people focus only on abs, and they think the key to a six-pack is to do as many sit-ups as possible. I love the plank, even though it's a yoga pose, because it's one of the most basic core exercises and is very effective. A lot of dudes think yoga is for "girls," but it has many benefits for everyone (yes, even if you're a bodybuilder). The extra hip rotation adds a degree of difficulty and helps widen the area of muscles worked during this exercise.

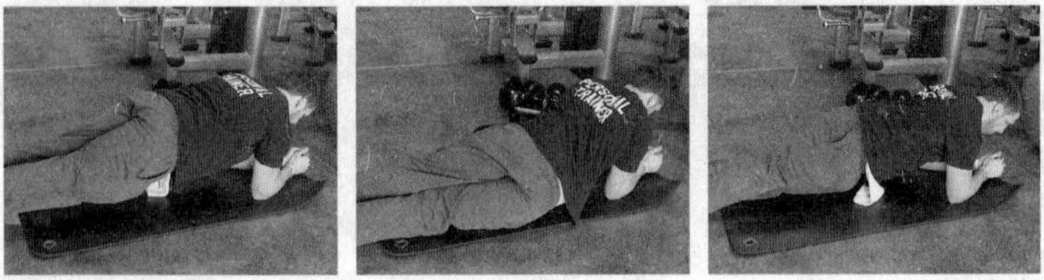

STEP 1 **Lie face down on a floor mat, resting on your forearms.**

STEP 2 **Push off the floor, raising yourself up onto your toes and resting on your elbows.**

STEP 3 **Concentrate on keeping your back flat, in a straight line from head to heels. Tilt your pelvis and contract your abdominals to prevent your rear end from sticking up in the air and your middle from sagging.**

STEP 4 **Rotate to one side by bringing one of your hips to touch the floor.**

STEP 5 **Return to the center position.**

STEP 6 **Rotate to the other side by bringing the other hip to the floor. Repeat.**

Side Planks with "Thread the Needle"

The side plank is another essential core exercise, reaching different muscles than a traditional plank. This exercise focuses on the obliques, hips, lower back, and "love handle" area. Being a guy, I get a lot of stares doing this one, since most guys in the gym are working some kind of ab-cruncher machine. The "thread the needle" motion adds an extra degree of difficulty to traditional side planks. This supplemental motion has many benefits, such as widening the area worked during the exercise—specifically, the motion helps to strengthen the small stabilizer muscles and improve balance.

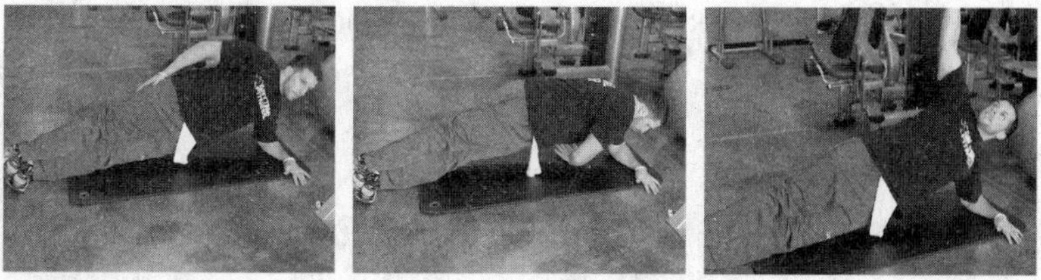

STEP 1 **Lie on your left side with your body straight, one foot on top of the other, but angled up from the hip to the shoulder. Support yourself with your left arm, bent 90 degrees at the elbow (your hand and forearm, flat on the floor, pointing directly in front of you). Rest your right arm on your right leg.**

STEP 2 **Push your midsection up so that only your left foot, hand, and forearm are in contact with the floor.**

STEP 3 **When you're in the correct position, the space left between you and the floor should form a triangle. Try not to let your hip sag and touch the floor.**

STEP 4 **Extend your right arm straight up (perpendicular to your body); then use that same arm to push through the triangular hole created by this position. Bring that arm back until it's completely extended away from your body. Repeat.**

STEP 5 **Switch sides and repeat.**

WORKOUTS

This appendix offers four workouts that combine exercises to strengthen the chest/back, legs/shoulders, biceps/triceps, and abs/core. For each exercise included, I offer three levels of difficulty. Begin where you feel comfortable and gradually work up to "The Breakthrough" level.

Within each workout, I specify how many reps and sets I do. Typically, I like to do my workouts as supersets—in other words, do two different exercises back to back with minimal or no rest between sets. This is great because you get the benefits of resistance training and cardio all in one.

I always start my workout with a warm-up, which can be anything from walking, biking, jumping, or running in place for a few minutes.

Chest/Back

Exercise 1: Push-Ups

With your body prone, place your hands on the floor so that they're about shoulder width apart. Rise up onto your toes so that all of your body weight is on your hands and feet. Bring your body into a straight line and keep it that way throughout the exercise. Bend your elbows and lower your chest toward the floor. Once your elbows bend slightly beyond 90 degrees, push off the floor again and extend your arms so that you return to starting position.

THE BEGINNING **As listed above, but with your legs resting on a stability ball (around hip level), which will provide less weight/resistance on your arms and shoulders when doing the push-up.**

THE BALANCE **As listed above.**

THE BREAKTHROUGH **As listed above, but with one hand on a medicine ball and the other on the floor.**

Exercise 2: Pull-Ups

Grip the pull-up bar with palms facing away from you. Extend your arms all the way and hang from the bar. Pull your body up without a swinging motion until your chin reaches above the bar. Then lower yourself back to the starting position.

THE BEGINNING **As listed above, using a chair or an "assisted" pull-up machine for support.**

THE BALANCE **As listed above.**

THE BREAKTHROUGH **As listed above, but with a 1-count on the way up and a 3-count on the way down.**

Here are the sets and reps I do for these first 2 exercises: 2 push-ups/1 pull-up, 4 push-ups/2 pull-ups, 6/3, 8/4, 10/5. Rest for 60 seconds and repeat 3 times.

Exercise 3: Dumbbell Flies

Grasp two dumbbells. Lie flat on a bench or lie on a stability ball with your knees bent. Support dumbbells above your chest, your arms slightly bent. With palms facing each other, open your arms from your shoulder joints, until your arms are parallel to the ground. Then contract the chest muscles by closing your arms to the starting position until the dumbbells touch back together. Repeat.

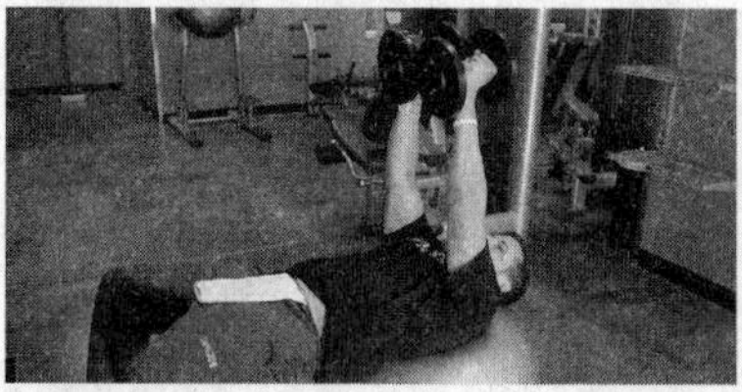

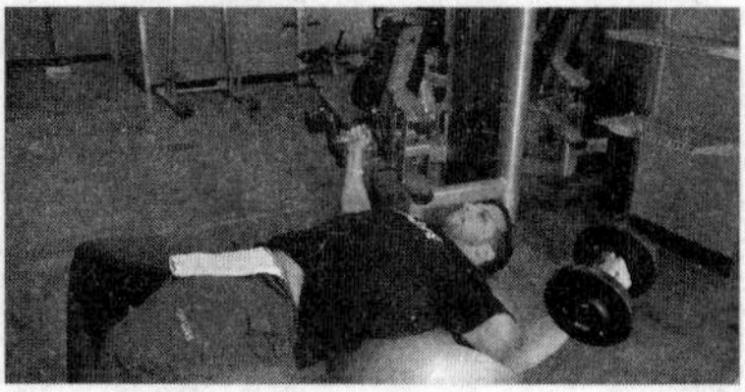

THE BEGINNING **As listed above, but with a light weight.**

THE BALANCE **As listed above, but with a pulse at the bottom.**

THE BREAKTHROUGH **As listed above, but with a 3-count on the way down and a 1-count on the way up.**

Exercise 4: Bent-over Rows

With feet shoulder width apart and knees slightly bent, bend over until your chest comes close to parallel with the floor. With dumbbells in hands and arms completely extended toward the floor, pull one dumbbell up to your side until it makes contact with your ribs or until your upper arm is just beyond horizontal. Return that arm to full extension, the shoulder stretched downward. Now pull the other arm up and back down.

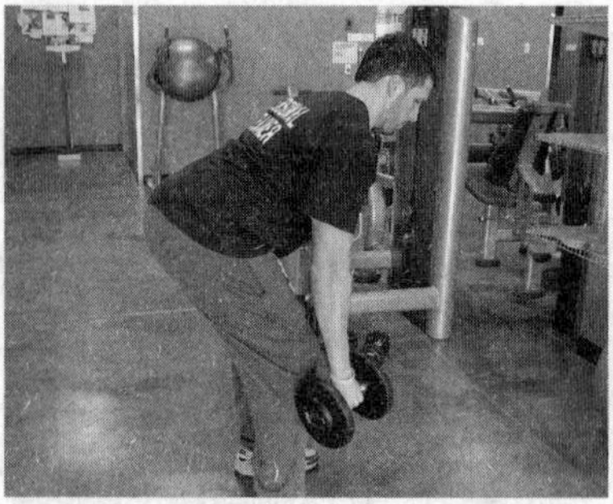

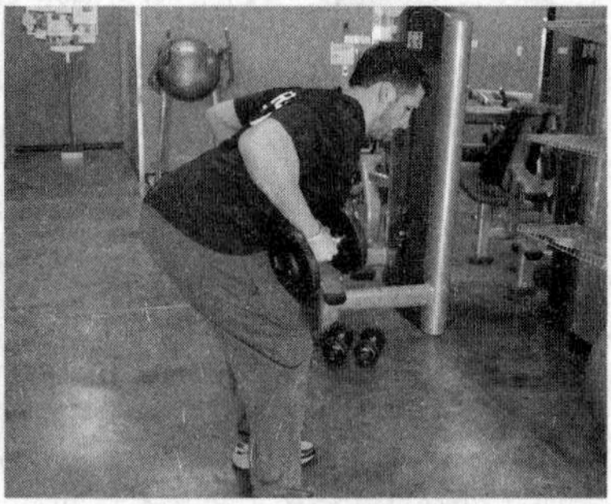

THE BEGINNING **As listed above, but with a light weight.**

THE BALANCE **As listed above, but on one foot with a slight pulse at the top.**

THE BREAKTHROUGH **As listed above, but on one foot with a 1-count on the way up and 3-count on the way down.**

Here are the sets and reps I do for exercises 3 and 4: exercise 3, 15 reps; exercise 4, 15 reps each arm. Repeat this superset 3 times with minimal to no rest in between.

Exercise 5: Dumbbell Bench Presses

Lie on your back on a stability ball with knees bent so that your body is parallel to the floor. With arms perpendicular to your body and bent upward at the elbow, hold the dumbbells out to the side. Press both dumbbells up until arms are extended. Lower dumbbells to the sides of your upper chest until a slight stretch is felt in the chest or shoulders.

THE BEGINNING **As listed above, but with a light weight.**

THE BALANCE **As listed above, but doing one arm at a time.**

THE BREAKTHROUGH **As listed above, but doing one arm at a time with a 1-count on the way up and a 3-count on the way down.**

Exercise 6: Dumbbell Deadlifts

Stand straight up, feet shoulder width apart, with dumbbells resting in your hands just in front of you, your arms fully extended downward. Slowly lower the dumbbells while keeping your back straight (though angled forward), chest out, and butt back until the dumbbells go below the kneecaps. Return to a fully standing position while keeping the dumbbells close to your body.

THE BEGINNING **As listed above, but with a light weight.**

THE BALANCE **As listed above, but with a barbell instead of dumbbells, and starting from the floor and coming all the way up and back down to the floor again for each rep.**

THE BREAKTHROUGH **As listed above, but with a barbell instead of dumbbells, and starting from the floor and coming all the way up and back down to the floor again for each rep, with a 1-count on the way up and a 3-count on the way down.**

Here are the sets and reps I do for exercises 5 and 6: exercise 5, 12 reps each arm; exercise 6, 12 reps. Repeat this superset 3 times with minimal to no rest.

Legs/Shoulders

Exercise 1: Dumbbell Squats

Stand with your feet shoulder width apart and with dumbbells in hands, resting at your sides. As you lower your body to a squat, stay back on your heels, keeping your chest out, back straight, and butt back. Go down until your thighs are parallel to the floor and come back up in the same motion.

THE BEGINNING **As listed above, but leaning your back against a stability ball (positioned between you and the wall), with a light weight or no weight.**

THE BALANCE **As listed above, but with a light barbell on the shoulders (right behind the neck) instead of dumbbells.**

THE BREAKTHROUGH **As listed above, but with a light barbell on the shoulders (right behind the neck) and doing jumping squats.**

Exercise 2: Dumbbell Military Presses

Stand with feet shoulder width apart and hold dumbbells above your shoulders, your arms extended out and then bent upward at a 90-degree angle. Raise the dumbbells straight above your head until your arms are fully extended, then bring them back down to the starting position.

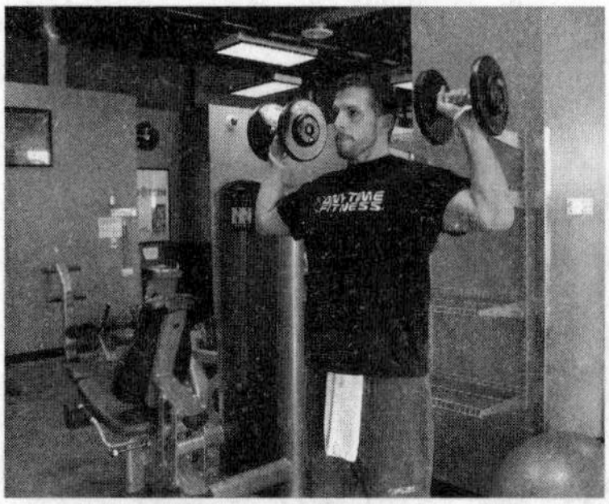

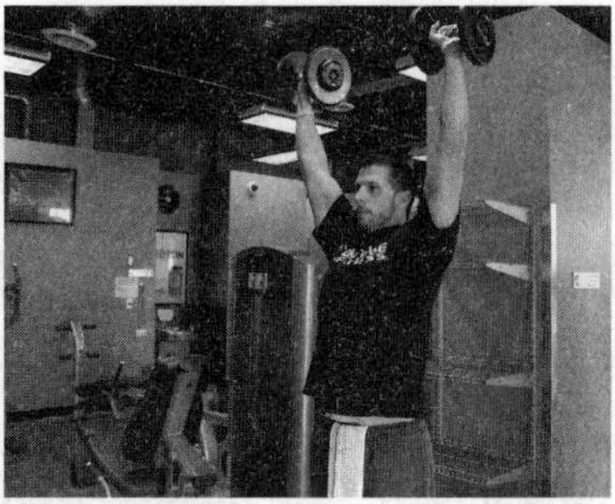

THE BEGINNING **As listed above, but with a light weight.**

THE BALANCE **As listed above, but on one foot.**

THE BREAKTHROUGH **As listed above, but on one foot, doing only one arm at a time.**

Here are the sets and reps I do for exercises 1 and 2: exercise 1, 15 reps; exercise 2, 12 reps. Repeat this superset 3 times with minimal to no rest in between.

Exercise 3: Lunges

Stand with one foot way out in front of you and the other back behind you with the back foot up on your toes. Go straight down, with back straight, until your front thigh is parallel to the floor, making sure that your front knee doesn't go in front of your front toes, then come back up to starting position.

THE BEGINNING **As listed above, but with light dumbbells hanging by your side.**

THE BALANCE **As listed above, but with the back foot up on a bench.**

THE BREAKTHROUGH **As listed above, but with light dumbbells and doing jumping lunges.**

Exercise 4: Side Dumbbell Raises

Stand with feet shoulder width apart and with light dumbbells resting by your sides, your arms hanging naturally. Bring both dumbbells up to the side until they're shoulder height, with arms completely extended away from your body. Slowly lower them to the starting position.

THE BEGINNING **As listed above, but with light dumbbells.**

THE BALANCE **As listed above, but on one foot.**

THE BREAKTHROUGH **As listed above, but on one foot, one arm at a time, with a pulse at the top.**

Here are the sets and reps I do for exercises 3 and 4: exercise 3, 12 reps each leg; exercise 4, 12 reps. Repeat this superset 3 times with minimal to no rest in between.

Exercise 5: Step-Ups

Stand in front of a bench, low chair, or you can use your home stairs. Step up with one leg, then use your foot that is on the step to push your other leg up until both feet are on the bench/chair/stair. Step down with the first foot leading. Then repeat, alternating feet.

THE BEGINNING **As listed above, but with light or no weight and on a smaller step/bench.**

THE BALANCE **As listed above, but with a knee raise added after the step up with the opposite leg.**

THE BREAKTHROUGH **As listed above, but doing jumping alternating step-ups.**

Exercise 6: Hand Step-Ups with Plank

Place a low step or a chair up against a wall for stability. Get in push-up position on the floor, facing that wall with the step/chair in front of you. Put one hand flat on the seat of the step/chair and return that hand immediately to the floor; now do the other hand (keeping your body in a straight line).

THE BEGINNING **As listed above, but doing it on your knees at a slow pace.**

THE BALANCE **As listed above.**

THE BREAKTHROUGH **As listed above, but doing it at a fast pace for at least 45 seconds per set.**

Here are the sets and reps I do for exercises 5 and 6: exercise 5, 15 each leg; exercise 6, 30 seconds at a fast pace. Repeat this superset 3 times with minimal to no rest in between.

Biceps/Triceps

Exercise 1: Chin-Ups

Grip the chin-up bar with palms facing you. Extend your arms all the way and hang from the bar. Pull your body up (without a swinging motion), using primarily your biceps, until your chin reaches above the bar. Return to the starting position.

THE BEGINNING **As listed above, but using a chair or an "assisted" pull-up machine for support.**

THE BALANCE **As listed above.**

THE BREAKTHROUGH **As listed above, but with a 1-count on the way up and a 3-count on the way down.**

Exercise 2: Dips

Sit on a chair with your hands on the edge a bit out from your hips. Walk your body away from the chair so that you're holding yourself up with your arms, and your feet are about shoulder width apart, giving you extra support. Go straight down until your arms form a 90-degree angle (keeping your elbows in and your back straight). Then return up to the starting position.

THE BEGINNING **As listed above, but with an "assisted" dip machine for support.**

THE BALANCE **As listed above.**

THE BREAKTHROUGH **As listed above, but with extra weight on your lap and with a pulse at the bottom.**

Here are the sets and reps I do for these first 2 exercises: exercise 1, 12 reps; exercise 2, 12 reps, then hold upright position for 10 seconds, then 12 more reps. Repeat this superset 3 times with minimal to no rest in between.

Exercise 3: Dumbbell Curls

Stand with feet shoulder width apart while holding dumbbells in hands. Let the weights hang in front of you with palms facing away from your body. While keeping your back straight, bring dumbbells up in the curve of a D-shaped motion, using your biceps. At the top, squeeze/flex the biceps. Return back down in the same D-shaped arc.

THE BEGINNING **As listed above, but with a light weight.**

THE BALANCE **As listed above, but on one foot.**

THE BREAKTHROUGH **As listed above, but on one foot, one hand at a time, with a pulse at the bottom.**

Exercise 4: Dumbbell Kickbacks

Stand holding dumbbells close to your body with elbows bent. Bend over so that your chest and upper arms are almost parallel to the floor. Extend your arms until they're straight (in other words, pointing behind you, because of your bent body), flex the triceps when arms are fully extended, then bring the arms back to the starting body-bent position.

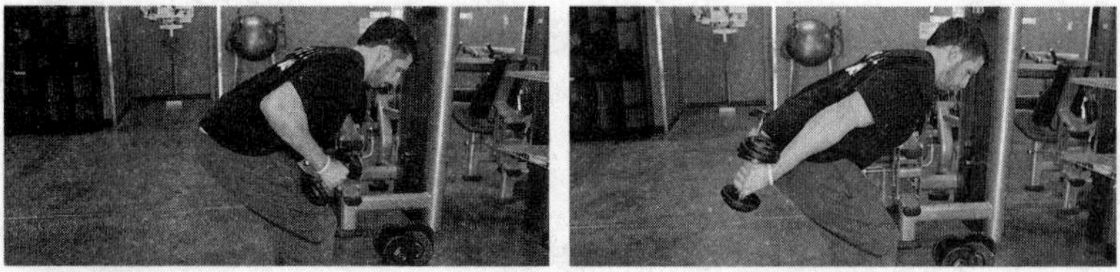

THE BEGINNING **As listed above, but with a light weight.**

THE BALANCE **As listed above, but on one foot.**

THE BREAKTHROUGH **As listed above, but on one foot, one hand at a time, with a pulse at the top.**

Here are the sets and reps I do for exercises 3 and 4: exercise 3, 15 reps each arm; exercise 4, 15 reps each arm. Repeat this superset 3 times with minimal to no rest in between.

Exercise 5: Hammer Curls

Stand with feet shoulder width apart. Holding dumbbells, let your arms hang by your sides with palms facing in toward your body. Bring one arm to a 90-degree angle pointing in front of you. Keeping your back straight, bring the other hand up and forward in the curve of a D-shaped motion, using your biceps. At the top, squeeze/flex the biceps and return back down in the same D-shaped arc. Switch sides and hold the other arm at a 90-degree angle while curling the second arm.

THE BEGINNING **As listed above, but with a light weight.**

THE BALANCE **As listed above, but on one foot.**

THE BREAKTHROUGH **As listed above, but on one foot, with a pulse at the bottom.**

Exercise 6: Triceps "Skull Crushers"

Lie down with your back on a stability ball, knees bent as needed, so that your body is parallel to the floor. Bring dumbbells straight up above your head with arms extended and palms facing each other. Bend your arms to 90 degrees so that the dumbbells reach your forehead on both sides. (Don't actually hit your head; just get close!) Return arms to extended position.

THE BEGINNING **As listed above, but with a light weight.**

THE BALANCE **As listed above, but with a pulse at the bottom.**

THE BREAKTHROUGH **As listed above, but with a 3-count on the way down and a 1-count on the way up.**

Here are the sets and reps I do for exercises 5 and 6: exercise 5, 12 reps each arm; exercise 6, 15 reps. Repeat this superset 3 times with minimal to no rest in between.

Abs/Core

I like to include core exercises in all my workouts. Sometimes I'll work them in between supersets, and other times I'll just do them at the end.

Exercise 1: Planks

Lie face down on a floor mat, resting on your forearms. Push off the floor, raising yourself up onto your toes and resting on your elbows. Concentrate on keeping your back flat, in a straight line from head to heels. Tilt your pelvis and contract your abdominals to prevent your rear end from sticking up in the air and your middle from sagging.

THE BEGINNING	**As listed above, but done on knees instead of on toes.**
THE BALANCE	**As listed above, but with a slight toe raise (meaning that you're pushing yourself slightly forward and back) during the exercise.**
THE BREAKTHROUGH	**As listed above, but on one foot, holding the other foot 6 inches off the floor.**

Do 3 sets of 30–45 seconds.

Exercise 2: Side Planks

Lie on your left side with your body straight, one foot on top of the other, but angled up from the hip to the shoulder. Support yourself with your left arm, bent 90 degrees at the elbow (your hand and forearm, flat on the floor, pointing directly in front of you). Rest your right arm on your right leg. Push your midsection up so that only your left foot, hand, and forearm are in contact with the floor. When you're in the correct position, the space left between you and the floor should form a triangle. Try not to let your hip sag and touch the floor. Then roll over and repeat the process on your right side.

THE BEGINNING **As listed above, but holding for only 10 seconds.**

THE BALANCE **As listed above, but with a slight wiggle at the hips, rotating back and forth for at least 30 seconds.**

THE BREAKTHROUGH **As listed above, but with a repeated "thread the needle" motion with your free arm (see page 215).**

Do 3 sets of 30 seconds on each side.

Exercise 3: Sunrise/Sunsets

Lie flat on your back on a mat with your arms and legs completely extended, forming a long horizontal line. Grasp a stability ball in your hands. Bring your arms, with stability ball, and your legs up until they meet in the middle. Then pass the ball from your hands to your feet, squeezing the ball between your feet to hold on. Lower your legs and arms simultaneously until they're almost parallel with the floor. Bring both arms and legs back up again and pass the ball back from feet to hands. Repeat this process.

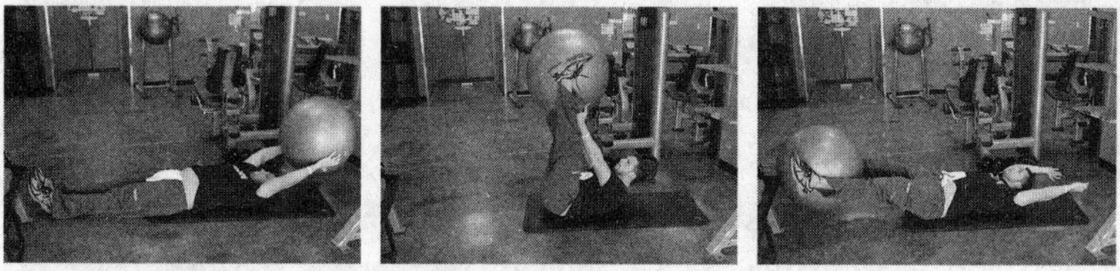

THE BEGINNING — **As listed above, but with no stability ball.**

THE BALANCE — **As listed above, but allowing the ball to touch/tap the floor.**

THE BREAKTHROUGH — **As listed above, but bringing head up to contract abs as arms/legs meet in the middle while not allowing the ball to touch the floor.**

Do 3 sets of 10 reps.

Exercise 4: Oblique Medicine Ball Passes

Sit on a mat with a medicine ball in your lap. Bring your feet up 6 inches off the floor, knees bent, and balance on your butt while leaning back slightly. (Your torso and upper legs will be in almost a V-shaped position.) Using both hands, touch the medicine ball to the floor on first one side of your body and then the other, maintaining the balance on your butt.

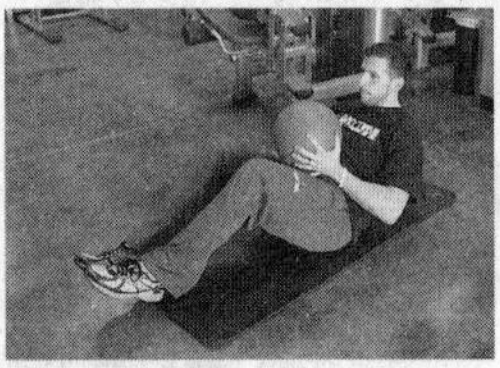
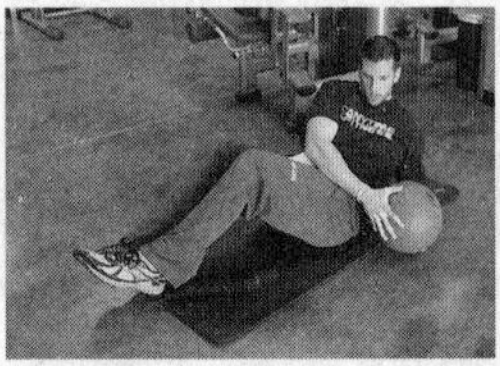
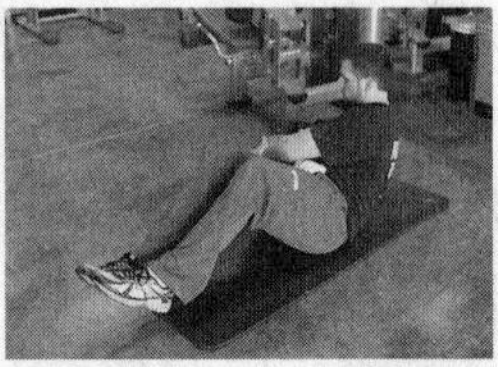

THE BEGINNING **As listed above, but with a light weight (or no) medicine ball and with feet resting on the floor.**

THE BALANCE **As listed above, at a fast pace.**

THE BREAKTHROUGH **As listed above, but with a heavier medicine ball at a fast pace for a longer period of time.**

Do 3 sets of 30 reps (15 each side).

Exercise 5: Wood Choppers

With a medicine ball, a single dumbbell, or a cable machine, start with the weight above your head and directly to the side of your body with arms extended. (It's okay if your head turns to that side of your body, too.) Without letting your hips twist, bring the weight down and across the front of you in an "ax" motion to about knee level; slightly bend the knees and twist your obliques during this motion. Bring your arms back up in a reverse motion, twisting your obliques back to starting position. Then change sides and repeat.

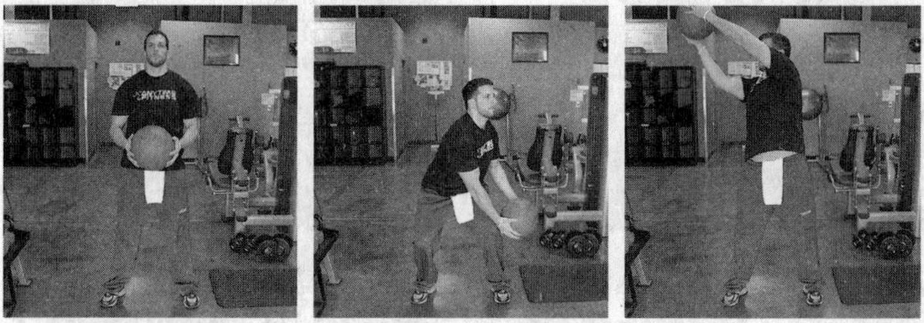

THE BEGINNING **As listed above, but with a light weight.**

THE BALANCE **As listed above, but with a heavier weight.**

THE BREAKTHROUGH **As listed above, but with a 1-count on the way down and a 3-count on the way up.**

Do 3 sets of 30 reps (15 each side).

Exercise 6: Hanging Leg Raises

Hang from a pull-up bar with palms facing away from you or inward toward each other. Without swinging your entire body, bend at the hips and bring your legs up slightly above parallel to the floor, knees slightly bent. At the top, tilt your pelvis upward, then bring legs back down slowly until you reach the starting position.

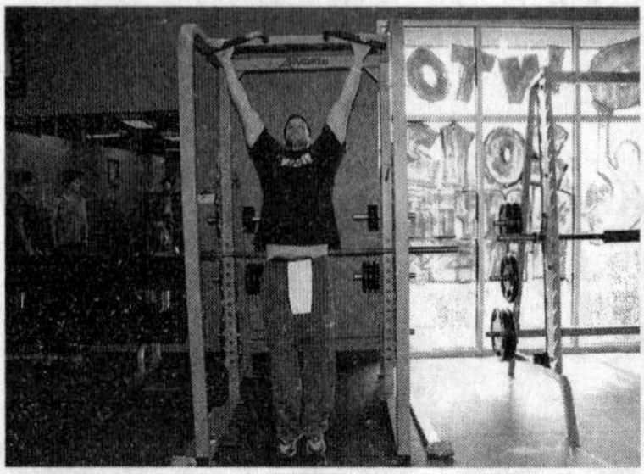

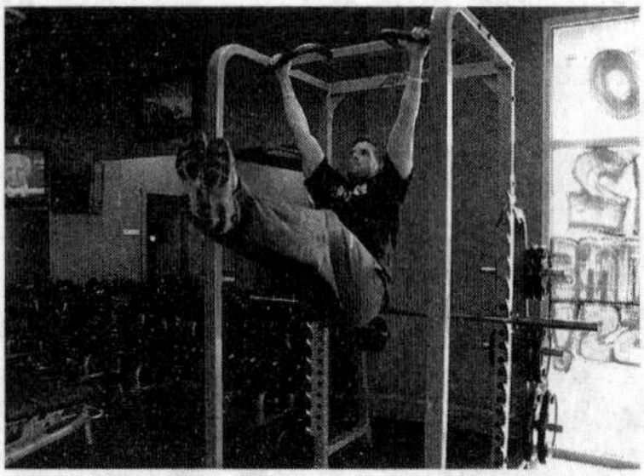

THE BEGINNING **As listed above, but using straps so that the weight is resting on your arms instead of just your hands, and bringing your knees to your chest instead of legs straight up.**

THE BALANCE **As listed above.**

THE BREAKTHROUGH **As listed above, but with a 1-count on the way up and a 3-count on the way down.**

Do 3 sets of 10 reps.

FIT2FAT2FIT

The Journey Continues

ONE YEAR LATER

Just when I think I have learned all there is to know about overcoming the emotional, mental, and physical struggles associated with gaining and losing weight, I get thrown new curveballs. I assumed that once I became fit again it would be easy to stay fit. After all, I was back to my "old" self. But like everything in life, you have to put effort in to get and maintain the results you want.

I enjoy exercising, but that doesn't mean that every run or workout is something I look forward to. No matter where we start, what our goals are, or whether we like to work out or not, we have to keep at it, keep pushing, and stay motivated.

Okay. More honesty. The cravings do not go away. Sure, they are easier to fight and less frequent now that a year has passed since I started my journey back to fit, but they are still there—just like the dreaded stretch marks on my love handles (thanks to the last week of my journey to fat): faded but always present. It's important to know that just like with any other addiction, once you reach your goal, you can't let your guard down. You must stay focused on the principles discussed in this book. Create new goals once you hit the ones you've made, maintain a support system, and schedule your breaks (cheat meals). This is the key to avoid relapsing into old habits.

Perhaps the most important lesson I've learned and

shared post-Fit2Fat2Fit is to not sweat the weight. At the end of the day, our scale doesn't tell us the whole picture. Yes, for me, I had to get back to 193 to "complete" my Fit2Fat2Fit journey, but what I didn't tell everyone is that I decided to gain a few pounds of lean muscle mass afterward. I felt a little too skinny even though I weighed about the same as I did pre-Fit2Fat2Fit. Just because we are losing weight or just because we are skinny doesn't mean that we're necessarily healthy. It's time to focus on becoming medically healthy first—weight loss and the beach body will be by-products of living this lifestyle over time.

So where am I a year after my journey of Fit2Fat2Fit? I kept the weight off, still have my six-pack, and still focus on making this a healthy lifestyle—*not* a diet!

I am excited to share some great new recipes and incredible Fit2Fat2Fit community success stories in the pages that follow. The members of the community continue to inspire each other every day, and Lynn and I are blessed to be a part of it.

Enjoy!

MY FIT2FAT2FIT JOURNEY

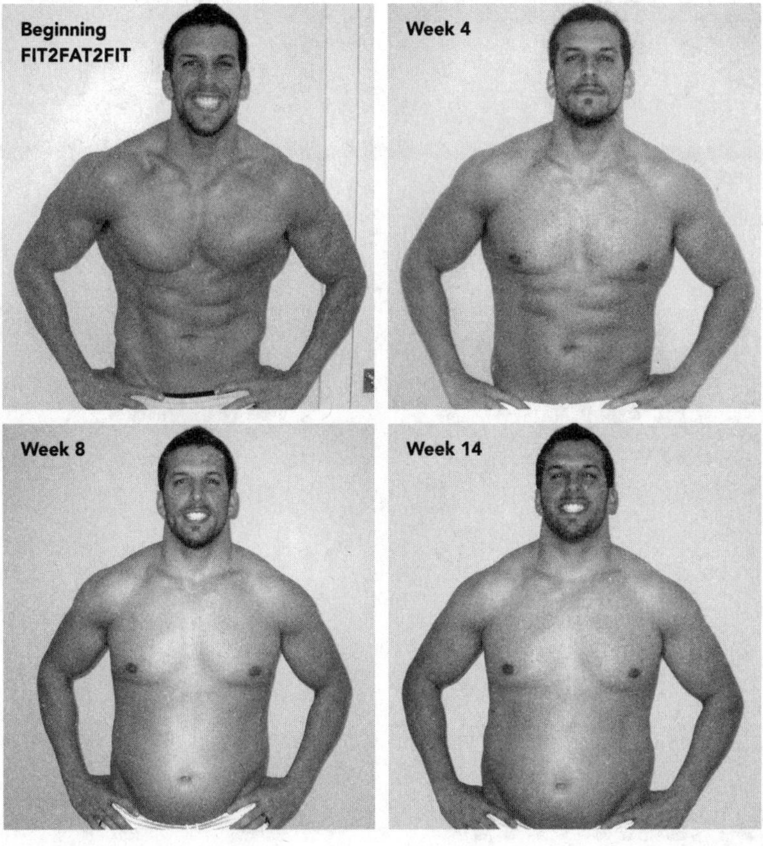

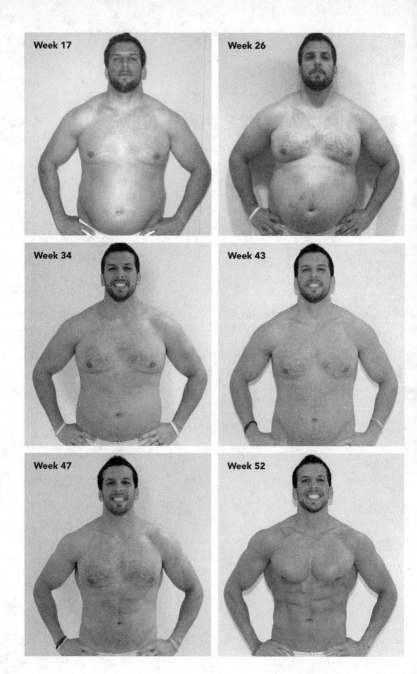

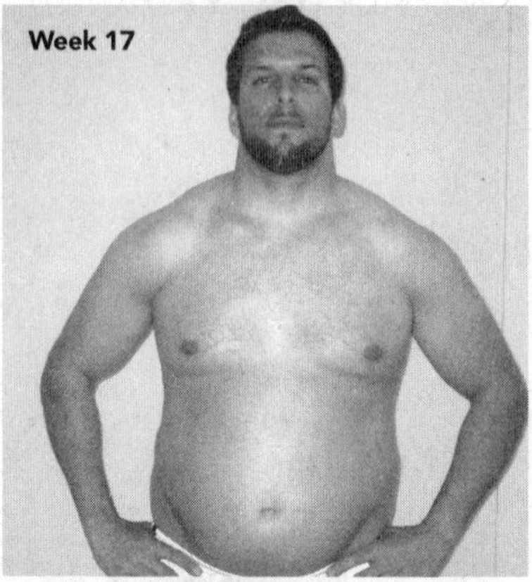
Week 17
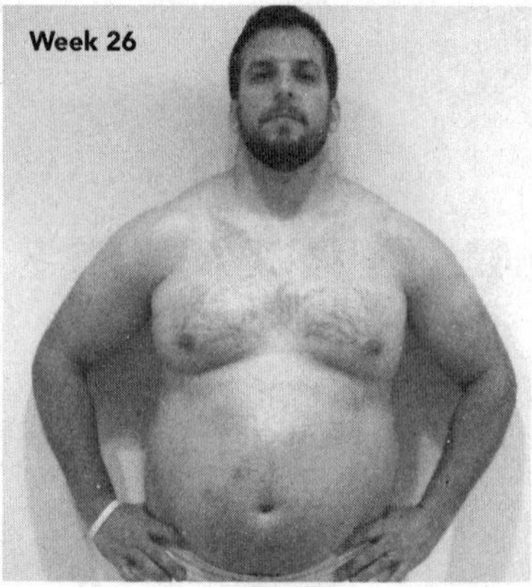
Week 26
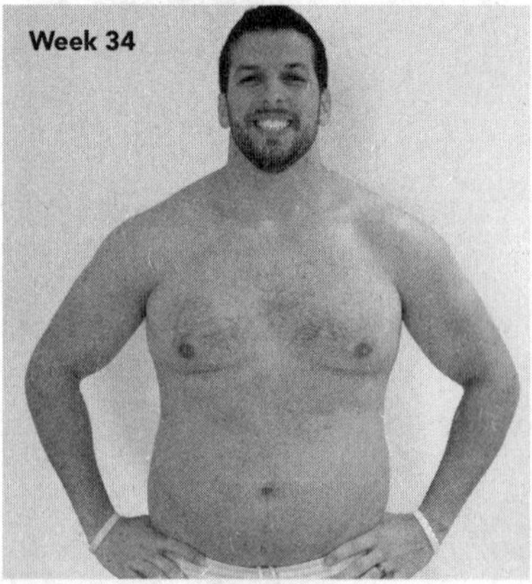
Week 34
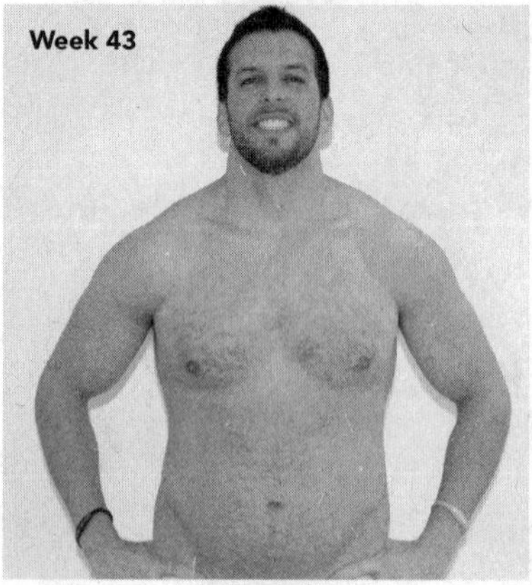
Week 43
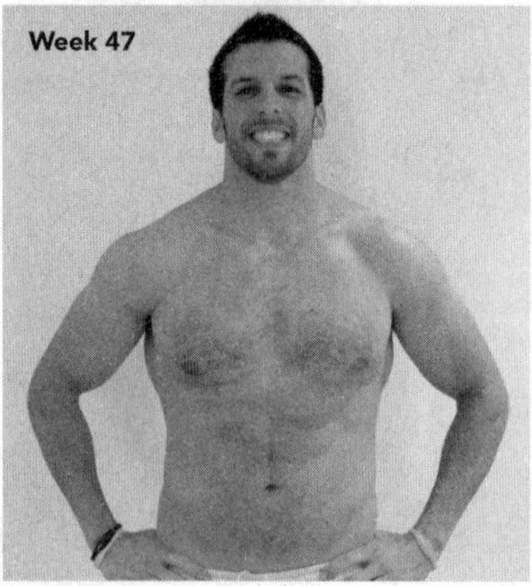
Week 47

Week 52

SIX NEW RECIPES

Butterfinger Protein Shake

Makes 1 serving

- ½ cup unsweetened almond milk
- ½ cup water
- 1 scoop vanilla Protein2Fit Natural Whey Isolate (or vanilla whey protein of your choice)
- 1 tablespoon sugar-free, fat-free butterscotch pudding mix
- 1 tablespoon sugar-free, fat-free chocolate pudding mix
- 1 tablespoon natural peanut butter
- 1 large handful spinach
- ¼ teaspoon xanthan gum (optional)
- 2–3 cups ice

Mix all ingredients in a blender and enjoy!

Cake Batter Protein Shake

Makes 1 serving

- ¾ cup unsweetened almond milk
- ¼ cup water
- 1 scoop vanilla Protein2Fit Natural Whey Isolate (or vanilla whey protein of your choice)

½ cap (or 3 drops) almond extract
½ cap (or 3 drops) butter extract
1 tablespoon sugar-free, fat-free vanilla pudding mix
2 packets xylitol (natural sweetener; this is optional)
5–10 ice cubes

Mix all ingredients in a blender and enjoy!

Pumpkin Protein Pancakes

Makes 2 servings Prep: 10 minutes Cook: 10 minutes

6 tablespoons egg whites
1 scoop vanilla Protein2Fit Natural Whey Isolate (or vanilla whey protein of your choice)
¼ cup pumpkin puree
1 packet xylitol or Stevia
¼ teaspoon cinnamon
¼ teaspoon nutmeg
¼ teaspoon butter extract
¼ teaspoon vanilla extract

Blend all ingredients together until mixed. Melt a small dab of coconut oil in a pan (low heat). Pour approximately ⅓ cup of mixture on skillet. Wait until the pancake starts to bubble and then flip with a spatula; cook other side. Makes about 4 medium-size pancakes.

Chicken Pizza

Makes 1 serving Prep: 15 minutes Cook: 10 minutes

1 boneless chicken breast
Dash of Italian seasoning
Dash of garlic powder
Dash of salt
1 tablespoon pizza sauce

½ ounce pepperoni

½ large fresh mushroom, thinly sliced

1 ounce cooked and crumbled Italian sausage

2 tablespoons minced green pepper

1 tablespoon minced red onion

Pound the chicken as thin as possible without tearing it. Season both sides of the chicken with the seasonings and place it on a foil-lined baking sheet. Spread the pizza sauce on the top of the chicken. Top the chicken with the rest of the ingredients. Bake at 400°F for 10 minutes or until chicken is cooked all the way through.

Red Cabbage Salad

Makes 10 servings   *Prep: 10 minutes*

2 cups red wine vinegar

1 cup olive oil

2 tablespoons crushed garlic

3 tablespoons Truvia

1 tablespoon salt

1 red cabbage, shredded

Cut the red cabbage into small bite-size pieces and place in a bowl. Mix in the rest of the ingredients and refrigerate.

Tip: This can be enjoyed right away, but it tastes better the next day after the ingredients have settled, especially if you mix the salad every three hours or so to allow the flavors to combine.

Sweet Potato Brownies

Makes 12 servings   *Prep: 40 minutes*   *Cook: 30–35 minutes*

1 sweet potato

3 eggs, whisked

¼ cup coconut oil, melted

½ cup Truvia

3 tablespoons coconut flour

2½ tablespoons unsweetened cocoa powder

¼ teaspoon baking powder

¼ teaspoon vanilla extract

¼ teaspoon cinnamon

Pinch of salt

Preheat your oven to 425°F. Use a knife or a fork to puncture the sweet potato before baking it for 25 to 30 minutes. Once your sweet potato is cooked all the way through, peel off its skin and mash it up in a bowl. Turn your oven down to 350°F. Now add in the Truvia, vanilla, whisked eggs, and coconut oil. Mix together. Now add in the coconut flour, cocoa powder, baking powder, cinnamon, and salt. Mix together. Grease an 8 x 8-inch glass baking dish with coconut oil and pour in the mixture. Bake for 30 to 35 minutes or until you can poke a toothpick in the middle and have it come out clean. Let it cool and enjoy.

SUCCESS IN THE FIT2FAT2FIT COMMUNITY

JC from Coquitlam, British Columbia, Canada

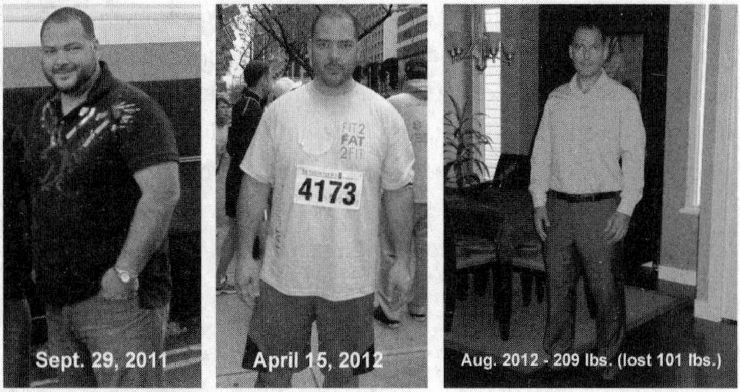

JC, Before and After

I don't have an emotional story on how I got to where I was, nor do I turn to food to make me feel better; I just loved to eat—the wrong foods, unfortunately. My Chilean background doesn't help either; we South Americans love our asados (BBQs)!

Over the last 10 years, my weight has been steadily climbing, and even though I had made attempts to losing weight,

I always found myself gaining it back. I was always left pondering several months later, What if I had stuck to it? Where would I be now?

At my heaviest, I was about 310 pounds and still somewhat active, but my weight was always holding me back from enjoying my favorite activities to the fullest. I scuba dive, hike, and ski, and I've always wanted to get into mountain biking, but being over 300 pounds kept me on the sidelines. After seeing some pictures of myself last summer and realizing I was dreading going to the doctor only to find out that I might be diabetic and have to go on medication or something even worse, I realized that I had to do something immediately.

I began my journey back to fit at the end of September 2011, and until I found your website in October, I had already lost 13 lb. Let me tell you—stumbling upon your site was one of the best things that could have happened to me. So now I have lost about 73 lb. WOW!

What a difference it has made. I sleep better, I barely snore, and now my wife doesn't have to wear earplugs. I feel great, I can ski better, my balance and flexibility have improved, and most importantly, I feel healthy. My only problem now is that I have to buy a whole new wardrobe.

I ran in the Vancouver Sun Run (10 km) representing Team Drew, and my time was 59 minutes; before, I would have died running around the block. If I had to sum up this journey in one word, I would say it has been "liberating." I cannot thank you guys enough for showing us the path to a healthier lifestyle.

Susie from Boise, Idaho

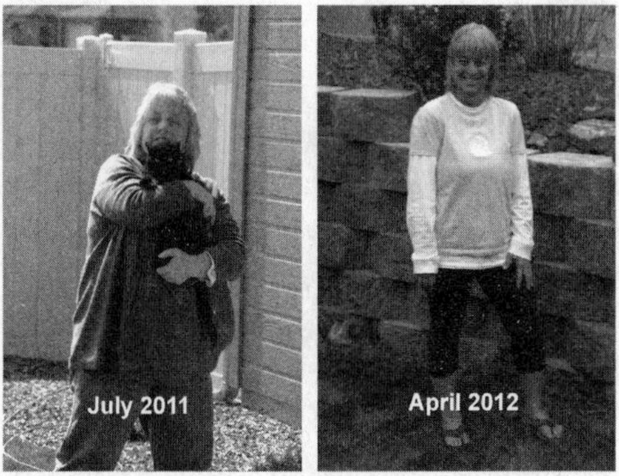

Susie, Before and After

My story may be different than others who have been spotlighted. I've eaten natural/organic foods for more than two decades. I didn't get fat by eating the standard American diet of high-calorie, processed foods and sugary sodas, which offer little or no nutrition. I was an emotional eater who didn't understand portion control, ate too many carbohydrates, and was addicted to natural ice cream.

Just like Drew became addicted to Cap'n Crunch cereal, brands like Ben & Jerry's and Starbucks were always in easy reach in my freezer. Add in a seven-year journey as a widow with two teenagers, and I can see why I got and stayed fat.

I can't blame anyone but myself. I put the food in my own mouth; I didn't exercise; I no longer knew what a healthy portion was; I consistently ate late at night—nearly every night. This is where my story begins. It's not where it ends.

My Fat2Fit journey began July 6, 2011. A couple weeks before, my sister called and shared the news of my nephew's upcoming wedding in May 2012. I had an immediate reaction of happiness mixed with dread. I broke out in a cold sweat: weddings translate to lots and lots of pictures.

Like Drew said, cameras don't lie. And I didn't look good. I certainly didn't look healthy or fit. I took my blood pressure. The numbers were shocking. I knew I wasn't healthy, but I realized at that moment that even though I had become comfortable with my increasing weight over the past years, my body was telling me just how unhealthy I had become.

I decided I wouldn't weigh myself; I knew the number on the scale would deter me from even starting any exercise. I measured myself instead. My initial numbers provided a second wake-up call. Just how had I let myself get so out of control? The real turning point for me was in early July. I'm embarrassed to write the next sentence: after 9 P.M., I consumed three entire pints of ice cream over three consecutive nights. I mindlessly ate one spoonful after another. I was shocked when my spoon hit the bottom of the pint the first night and I discovered the pint was empty. Yet I repeated the same exercise in emotional eating the next night and then once again on the following night. I woke up on the third night coughing and choking and feeling like I was suffocating. At first I thought I had a nightmare. What I realized right then was I was actually living a health nightmare! That lack of air had never happened before. I experienced sleep apnea for the first time in my life.

Upon waking the next morning, I was determined to change my life. I put on comfortable old sweats and a T-shirt and started—simply walking around my neighborhood. I had two kids at college at the same time, so I didn't want to pay to go to a gym. That first day, I looked at my pedometer: not even a tenth of a mile, and I was huffing and puffing like an old steam engine going uphill. Yet I continued. I felt ridiculously better after only 10 days. At that point it was no longer about the upcoming pictures at the wedding but how much better I felt. I told myself, "If you did it yesterday, there's no reason you can't do it again." That became my mantra.

I started a spreadsheet on my computer to chart my progress. Days turned into weeks, weeks into months. I measured myself on the last day of the month to chart my progress. I competed against my best mileage and even did 13.2 miles in one day.

Neighbors remarked how dedicated I was, and that inspired me to keep going—no matter how long it took to get fit. The time a neighbor applauded from his driveway as I walked by encouraged me even more. Then a miracle happened.

In October 2011, I heard about Drew and his Fit2Fat2Fit journey. I thought he was a bit crazy! Who intentionally puts his health on the line to inspire other people to get fit? From Drew and Lynn, I learned the importance of core exercises, drinking a 16 oz. glass of water upon waking, and consistent exercise every day.

I continued to walk—no matter how cold or windy it was or what excuse my mind offered up to me to stop. I had undergone such a physical change that I got numerous comments from acquaintances telling me they didn't recognize me. That inspired me further.

I challenged my son to an exercise contest. We did wall sits, push-ups, and planks. I was his once-out-of-shape, obese mom doing the same exercises on the floor as him! I realized I had transformed myself in only 9–10 months.

In mid-March, I got caught in the rain after grocery shopping and ran to my car parked at the end of the lot. It was a cats-and-dogs kind of rain, and I ran for the sheer joy of running. I felt the rain splatter on my face but didn't feel my heart pounding at all. I lifted my head up to the heavens as my face turned into one huge grin. It was at that moment that I realized I had fulfilled what I hoped for at the beginning of this journey: I had become healthy and fit. I'm so grateful to Drew and Lynn. I do know if I was to complete a list of the top 10 people who have had the most influence on my life, their names would be included. I'm here to tell you every mile walked, every core exercise pushed through, every excruciating wall sit, every kettlebell lifted, every ache and pain endured, and every time I made the right choice on food have been worth it. For me, it has nothing to do with the number on some scale; it has everything to do with how you feel.

ACKNOWLEDGMENTS

I'd like to dedicate this book to my three girls . . . my amazing, beautiful wife, Lynn, for her unconditional support and for putting up with my snoring and laziness throughout my Fit2Fat stage, and my two beautiful daughters, Kale'a and Kiana. You three motivate me more than anyone, and without you this book would not have been possible.

Also, a special thanks to my family, friends, and amazing followers, who inspired me when the days were tough and reminded me of the purpose of this journey.

And to all of you for buying my book. For many of you, this is your first step in becoming healthy, and I'm humbled to be a part of that amazing journey!

Scan this code with your smartphone to be linked to bonus materials for *FIT2FAT2FIT* and other healthy living books and information.

You can also text keyword FAT2FIT to READIT (732348) to be sent a link to the mobile website.